S0-BEZ-136

MOVE IT!

*An Exercise and Movement Guide
for People with Parkinson's Disease*

Bensenville Community Public Library
200 S. Church Road
Bensenville, IL 60106

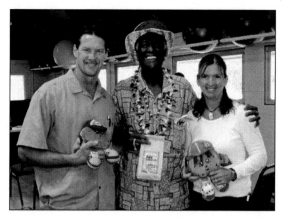

Kevin Lockette, physical therapist, author of
MOVE IT, with Wally Amos, narrator and Ginger
Lockette, physical therapist.

Also Available on DVD featuring Wally Amos as the narrator.

This DVD includes demonstrations of movement techniques, three levels
of exercise programs to simply follow along and much more! Parkinson's
Disease (PD) is a movement disorder that is unique. Due to this fact, it
was felt the video/DVD format is the best method to illustrate movement
techniques and exercise using people who suffer from PD.

To purchase DVD go to **www.parkinsonsmoveit.com** or send check
payable to Ohana Pacific Rehab for $24.00 plus $5.00 postage and
handling (for continental US orders) to:

MOVE IT (DVD)
Ohana Pacific Rehab Services

Ohana Pacific Rehab
354 Uluniu Street, Suite 404
Kailua, HI 96734

or call us at (808) 262-1118 to place your order.

NOTE: Physical disability with PD can vary greatly. Health and wellness are matters that require individual consideration. Readers should consult their physicians regarding their individual needs before engaging in an exercise program. This book is not intended to replace rehabilitation programs through the medical profession. It should be used as a guide to promote and maintain wellness in conjunction with the medical profession. Any application of the recommendations set forth in this book is at the readers' discretion and risk.

DEDICATION

To all Parkinson's Disease sufferers with whom I have had the pleasure and privilege to work with. Your courage and inner strength is truly inspiring.

To my wife, Ginger, and my children, Griffin and Hudson. Mahalo (Thank you) for your love and patience during my hours spent on this project.

Bensenville Community Public Library
200 S. Church Road
Bensenville, IL 60106

TABLE OF CONTENTS

PREFACE

Welcome to, *"MOVE IT! –An Exercise and Mobility Guide for People with Parkinson's Disease"*. This project was inspired by you- people with Parkinson's Disease (PD). I have seen many people with PD as a physical therapist and I have taught classes for PD support groups for years. To my amazement nearly every time, there were folks, both newly diagnosed or persons who had PD for 20+ years, who stated that they learned something that made a profound difference in their daily lives. I continued to teach and continued to get cards and phone calls of gratitude for the techniques that were taught-- "Thanks for teaching me 'the poor man's hula'. I can get out of being frozen so easily now.", "I use the imaginary poles when I have to get up at night and now I rarely fall!", "My exercise program gives me so much energy the next day I almost forget to take my meds.", "My friends comment on my posture. They say I look taller!", etc. My PD patients, friends, and caregivers have persistently encouraged me to pursue this project to bring this useful information to a wider audience. This book and companion video will share many non-conventional exercises and techniques that I have found helpful from working with persons with PD keep moving over the last 19 years. I have learned much from the wonderful PD patients I have had the privilege to work with over these many years. I will share many of their valuable insights in the following pages.

Exercise in conjunction with medication is one of the best things that you can do to counteract the negative physical effects of Parkinson's disease. If you are newly diagnosed or have longstanding PD, this book will give you guidelines for how to move more effectively despite your PD and how to stave off further physical decline. You will also find strategies and techniques that will help you everyday in remaining mobile while dealing with the physical symptoms of PD. Traditional or conventional exercise programs do not always carry-over well or meet the specific needs for those dealing with PD symptoms.

In Chapter One we will review the physical manifestations of Parkinson's so that we can better understand how to combat them. In Chapter Two, we will teach you mobility techniques that apply both scientific approaches of physical therapy as well as pragmatic solutions. In Chapter Three, we will review assistive devices for safer walking. In Chapter Four, we will look at not only fall prevention strategies, but also how to fall and what to do when you are on the floor. In Chapter Five, we will review many of the adaptive equipment devices that will help you maintain your independence. In Chapters Six through Ten we will teach you the principles of exercise and a series of exercise programs that are exclusively designed for Parkinson's Disease. In Chapter Eleven we will present the principles of stretching and a flexibility program designed to maintain independence and to avoid other musculo-skeletal injuries.

Let's get you started on this journey.

Kevin Lockette PT

ACKNOWLEDGEMENTS

This project could not be what it is without the assistance of many. Thank you so much for your contributions to this project:

CONTENT REVIEWERS: Melvin Yee M.D., Michicko Bruno M.D., Ginger Lockette PT, Jerry Ono PT, Beth Leever PT, Alison Aldcroft PT, Peggy Hill PT, Martin De Bueger PT, Arlene Ono OT, Jack Richardson, Lorraine Kent, Danielle Clark, Michael O'Conell, Katherine Kim, Carrie Vallo, Noreen Conlin.

CONTRIBUTING AUTHORS:
Melvin Yee M.D. Chapter One: About Parkinson Disease
Arlene Ono OT   Chapter Five: Adaptive Devices

PARTICIPANTS: Jack Richardson, Lorraine Kent, Josh Gianelli, Grace Takabayashi, Cindy Vasquez, Doug Smoyer, David Lerps

COVER ART WORK: Aaron Katagiri

CHAPTER ONE

About Parkinsons Disease

Melvin Yee M. D.

Before you start learning the mobility techniques and exercises, it is necessary to briefly review the possible physical symptoms of Parkinson's Disease so that we can teach you how to combat and stave off these symptoms through the techniques and exercises that will be presented throughout this book. We will also review what we understand about what causes Parkinson's and a bit about the treatment of the disease.

CAUSE

Parkinson's disease (PD) was first described by Dr. James Parkinson in "An Essay on the Shaking Palsy" in 1817. Most of PD starts in a part of the brain called the substatia nigra. This is located deep in the brain in a section called the midbrain. Substantia nigra means the Black Stuff. Scientists noticed that this black stuff was missing from the brains of patients who died with PD. In fact, Parkinson's was found to occur when about 80 % of the black stuff had disappeared. This black stuff was believed to be something extremely important.

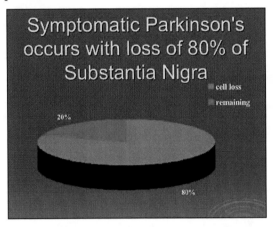

It turns out that the black stuff is a chemical called dopamine. Dopamine is required to control movement; low levels of dopamine are the primary reason for the motor symptoms in PD.

The cause of PD is not completely understood; however, researchers are studying possible environmental or genetic factors behind the disease. This may be easily understandable if you happen to be a neurologist or had a PhD in neurophysiology… But what does all of this mean in every day terms?

Think of the basal ganglia as a fine machine with cogs and wheels just like your mother's old sewing machine.

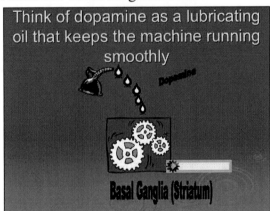

Your mother had to oil that machine to keep it running smoothly. Think of dopamine as a fine lubricating oil that keeps the machine directing the movement of your muscles running smoothly. Where did this fine lubricating oil come from? It had to come from a refinery before it was available.

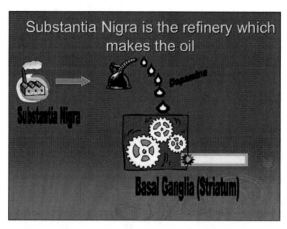

Think of the substantia nigra as the refinery that makes the fine lubricating oil dopamine. Dopamine keeps the machinery in the basal ganglia running well. If the refinery shuts down then not enough oil is made to keep the machinery running smoothly.

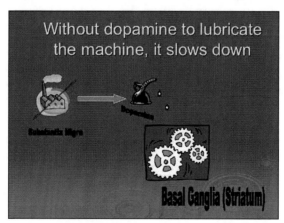

If the substantia nigra stops working then not enough dopamine is made to help the body keep the muscles running smoothly. That's when Parkinson's Disease occurs.

DEMOGRAPHICS

Over one million Americans, and an estimated six million people worldwide, currently live with PD. It is reported that there are nealy 50,000 new cases diagnosed each year and prevalence surveys have found that 35-42% of cases of the general population go undiagnosed. The average age of onset is approximately 62 years old; however, up to 10% of persons with PD are diagnosed before the age of 40. PD is rarely seen before the age of 30.

DIAGNOSIS

There is no definitive test available today to diagnosis PD; rather, it is diagnosed on the basis of clinical history and findings of a neurological exam. Parkinsonism is the term applied to a group of physical symptoms of resting tremors, slowness of movement (bradykinesia), rigidity of muscles, and instability of posture and walking. The presence of at least two of these cardinal signs is necessary for the definitive diagnosis of PD. The variety and severity of symptoms vary from person to person. Symptoms typically appear insidiously on one body part or side of the body but progress to affect the entire body over time.

CARDINAL PHYSICAL SYMPTOMS

It is important to understand the physical features of PD in order to plan an exercise program specifically designed to aid in decreasing or combating these symptoms. Let's take each symptom one at a time.

Resting Tremor

Resting tremors are by far the most recognizable of all PD features.

Tremors are seen in approximately 75% of PD cases. Tremors are evident at rest and decrease with purposeful movement. Tremors can initiate in one body part such as the fingers, hand, foot, arm, leg, jaw or tongue and are typically asymmetrical. It is not typical to see tremors in the head or neck. Tremors can increase with walking, stress, and anxiety; they usually disappear during sleep.

Rigidity

Rigidity is an involuntary increase in muscle tone that results in continuous resistance to passive movement. It has been described by some patients as internal resistance to movement. I have had other patients compare it to trying to move through mud. Rigidity superimposed with tremors results in a ratchet type of resistance to passive movement described as "cog-wheel" rigidity. It feels like a continuous catch-release when trying to passively move a limb (arm/leg).

Bradykinesia (Slowness of movement)/Freezing

Bradykinesia is a very significant feature of PD that affects all aspect of movement including walking, crossing the street, dressing, putting on shoes, bed mobility, getting out of a car, food preparation, eating, brushing teeth, etc. There can also be a progression from slow moving to having some difficulty initiating movement. One study suggests that step initiation correlates with sensory information from the basal ganglia. Since this sensory feedback loop is disturbed in PD, you may require external cues to achieve appropriate functional movement. The difficulty with initiating movement comes into play with changing directions with walking or turning corners. Freezing episodes can also occur. The freezing phenomenon is when you are truly frozen and virtually unable to move. Some people describe their freezing episodes as "feeling like my feet are glued to the floor." Many scenarios can trigger freezing episodes. Some common triggers include crossing thresholds, turning corners, surface changes such as carpet to multi-color or non-uniform tile patterns, as well as entering or exiting elevators and escalators.

Postural Instability

The loss of postural reflexes and the associated inability to make rapid postural corrections can also lead to declining gait and falls. Your reflexes and ability to catch yourself following loss of balance are either absent or too impaired to avoid a fall. If your balance gets offset backwards, you would basically fall like a cut tree. Essentially if your balance is offset, you may not be able to recover, so prevention is the key. Posture plays one of the most significant roles in both risk and prevention of falls. The more that you are able to keep your center of gravity over your base of support (your legs), the less likely you are to fall. For this reason, the suggested exercise programs presented later will be focused on posture and purposeful movements.

Medications

The treatment of PD requires many modalities. Exercise and medications are the two of the most beneficial strategies to assist you in staving off the physical symptoms of PD. This book will focus on mobility techniques and exercise. Before we get into the mobility techniques, let's briefly discuss some of the medications that are used to treat PD.

As I discussed earlier, if the Substantia Nigra stops working then not enough dopamine is made to help the body keep the muscles running smoothly. Levodopa (L dopa) is the building block from which the substantia nigra makes more dopamine.

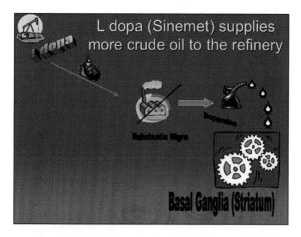

Supplying more L dopa to the body is like shipping more crude oil to the refinery where it will be made into the fine lubricating oil for keeping the machine running smoothly. Unfortunately L dopa can cause a lot of nausea.

Carbidopa/levodopa or Sinemet has an added ingredient carbidopa which makes the delivery of L dopa more efficient.

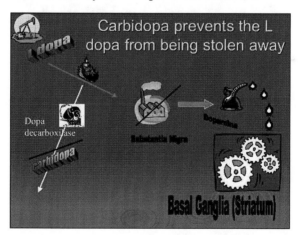

There are still some major side effects of carbidopa levodopa which you need to be aware of. These may include, nausea, intestinal upset, sleepiness, dizziness and, in some cases, confusion or hallucinations.

Sewing machine oil is not the only type of oil that you could use to lubricate your machine. You could go out, harpoon a whale, and make the blubber into oil. Likewise, Cabidopa/ Levodopa is not the only thing that can lubricate the basal ganglia.

Other drugs called the dopamine agonists (Mirapex® and Requip®), also work in the same way. Similarly these can have the very same side effects: nausea, GI upset, sleepiness, dizziness, and sometimes confusion or hallucinations. They may also cause swelling in the legs.

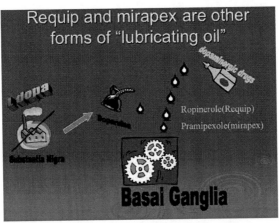

The Anticholinergics (artane or trihexiphenydyl and cogentin or benztropine)work down the line to keep the machine moving.

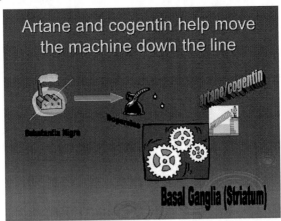

These drugs, however, must be used with great caution because of their risk of producing hallucinations, confusion, and worsening constipation.

Amantadine is another one of the older medications used for PD. It causes the basal ganglia to release more dopamine.

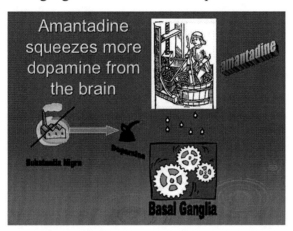

These days it is often used to treat dyskinesia, which can occur in more advanced cases of the disease. Dyskinesia occurs when the brain can't control its use of dopamine; the patient can have too much dopamine effect for his/her amount of movement. Any machine has to be able to dispose of the excess lubricating oil. In the basal ganglia there are two drains for dopamine known as MAO and COMT. By blocking MOA by use of selegeline (eldepryl®) or rasageline (azilect®) the amount of dopamine available to the basal ganglia can be increased. Similarly results may be obtained by blocking COMT by use of entacapone (comtan®).

Some patients can benefit from a new surgical technique called deep brain stimulation. A neurosurgeon uses a technique called stereotactic surgery to place a small wire deep into the brain. The wire is then hooked up to a small generator, much like a pacemaker, which sends electrical impulses into the target area of the brain.

The technique does not cure the patient with Parkinson's Disease but it can help. It lessens fluctuation of motor function and keeps a patient at his or her best active state for more time during the day. This procedure is not for everyone and does include the risks associated with surgery.

Now that you have a basic understanding of the physical symptoms of Parkinson's Disease and the common medications, you can learn the techniques and exercises presented in the following chapters that will assist you in combating and/or staving off these physical symptoms.

Note: *There is a host of other PD symptoms that do not involve mobility which will not be covered. These are out of the scope of the content focus in this book.*

CHAPTER TWO

Movement Challenges: Strategies & Tips to Keep You Moving

NO MORE AUTOMATIC PILOT

Prior to experiencing any PD symptoms, you did not have to think to move. You simply got up and walked, turned, lifted, twisted, ran, etc. You did not think about it at all. You simply relied upon your "automatic pilot." Well, with PD, your automatic pilot does not function well and may not work at all at times as you may experience "freezing episodes". In this chapter we are going to teach how to move consciously, after adding techniques and strategies to your bag of tricks to assist you in getting out of trouble when PD symptoms threaten your ability to move. We will help you establish your "personal trick." Most of you will find the greatest difficulty with movement during the "wearing off" periods of your medications. The practical strategies presented will assist you with your mobility, keep you out of trouble, and hopefully assist in preventing falls.

CONSCIOUS POSTURE & PURPOSEFUL MOVEMENT

The keys to moving more freely with PD are primarily conscious posture and purposeful movement. You now have to think to move. The trick is that you have to re-train yourself this way. At first this can be mentally fatiguing because you are not use to thinking about general movement; however, with practice, you will have the ability to maintain safe, effective mobility, and stave off or delay the physical effects of PD presented in Chapter One.

Strategies that I have found helpful are, first, to visualize the activity, whether it be walking, turning, standing, etc. Second, mentally plan the sequence of the activity you wish to achieve in defined steps. Third, completely finish each step of the sequence prior to starting the next step and lastly, complete the task or activity prior to starting the next one. This strategy forces purposeful, conscious movement. There are techniques and cues that will be presented later in this chapter that will assist you in keeping your movement "mindful."

❖ *Visualize*
❖ *Plan*
❖ *Sequence (one step at a time)*
❖ *Complete*

BLENDING STEPS OF A SEQUENCE

One common feature seen with PD is the blending of movement sequences. Blending is defined as starting step 1 but prior to completing step 1 you are already starting or "blending" in steps 2 & 3. An example is a simple transfer to a chair from standing. Blending occurs when you approach a chair, but before you complete the approach, you reach for the chair and start to turn and sit all at the same time. A better approach is to use auditory cues to break down and perform the sequences one at a time such as talking to yourself, "Approach chair, turn to square buttocks over chair, reach back for chair, then sit." Again, you can't rely on that old automatic pilot. You have to turn off the faulty automatic pilot, grab the wheel, and steer the plane, one step at a time. With practice, you can actually train yourself to move in this way and most likely avoid some falls.

One technique that is helpful to avoid blending is to focus on the destination. Walk up to the desired spot and make contact with your leg. An example would be approaching your bed. Focus on a spot on the bed where you wish to sit. Walk straight up until your leg makes contact with the bed. By doing this, you have at least eliminated premature reaching and turning before you are close enough to sit down.

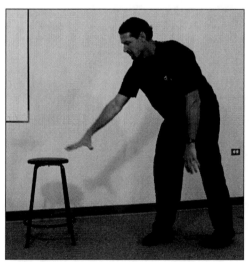

An example of blending of sequence by approaching, turning, and sitting at same time.

TIP : When turning corners or turning to sit down, plan out your steps so that you are conscious of what each foot is doing. Try not to pivot on one leg but rather take smaller steps. One problem with PD is that you will have a tendency to combine steps, so you have to consciously perform one step at a time when turning corners or when approaching a chair to sit. Below is an example of this. When you combine steps you will typically try to step, rotate your trunk, and pivot all at the same time, which can lead to freezing or falls; however, if you break it down to individual steps of a sequence, you can maintain good dynamic balance.

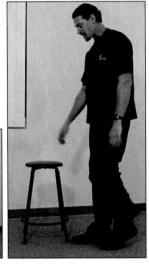
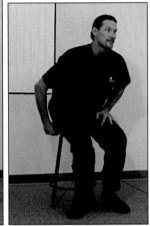
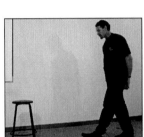

DARN THAT GRAVITY/ FORWARD POSTURING

Posture: Due to the physical symptoms of PD mentioned above, posture is nearly always affected and plays a huge role in how you walk and move in general. Typical posture changes include standing with your knees and hips bent with a rounded upper back, rounded shoulders, and a forward head. You will also typically see the arms tucked into the side of the body with the elbows flexed and hands/fingers curled in towards the body.

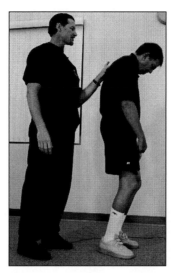

Shows rounded shoulders and forward head.
This posture places the muscles at a mechanical disadvantage
taking more energy to keep head up and promotes forward
posture which can impair your walking and balance.

This stooped posture has a huge impact. You know the drill. You stand up and gradually (or fairly immediately), gravity gets the best of you and you find yourself bending forward as though you are looking for change on the ground. When your center of gravity is in front of your base of support (your feet), your postural muscles are at a disadvantage. Your hip and back extensors have to work much harder to hold you up because your skeleton is no longer vertically stacked. Maintaining this flexed posture leads to fatigue and often back pain. This posture also increases the tendency to fall forward when walking or backward when trying to reach overhead while standing. In walking with this stooped posture, you are basically trying to catch up with your center of gravity; this can cause a rapid uncontrollable shuffling gait. I have even worked with a patient who couldn't control her gait once she started in the pattern and literally ran into the wall or a stable object in order to right herself.

Posture also affects your ability to perform activities of daily living. One of the first restrictions noticed is loss in shoulder range of motion (ROM) which impairs the ability to perform basic tasks such a dressing yourself and bathing. Understanding these typical PD postures is important, as your exercise program design will work to directly oppose these postures.

TIP: *When you are slumped, your skeleton is no longer mechanically stacked, which actually puts your muscles at a mechanical disadvantage; in other words, your muscles have to work harder to pull you up. You may cue your body by squeezing your shoulder blades together while straightening your knees and squeezing your buttock muscles. If you are having difficulty with standing, you can perform the posture correction of squeezing your shoulder blades when sitting as well. This will force your body to realign itself. Do this throughout the day. Your "automatic pilot" is not working so you have to consciously think to do this. You will, over time, try to re-engage your "postural muscles" through conscious thought, then maintain a more advantageous posture.*

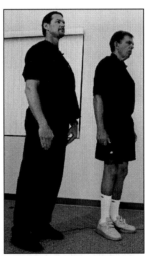

An example of self-conscious posture correction that can be performed throughout the day in both standing and sitting.

TIP: There are different postural shoulder braces on the market that are designed to decrease the rounded shoulder posture. I have had some success with these braces. The intent is to encourage activation of the scapular muscles throughout the day. Most of these braces have some elasticity so they give you support but without restricting your movement. Typically you wear it during the day, but take it off at night and during any exercise program for your upper body. Some of you may find that the constant cue of the brace during the day helps "retrain" your postural muscles by giving them a consistent reminder. In some cases, you can use the brace as a temporary means of training your posture and in other cases, you may choose to wear the brace indefinitely to give you a little extra help.

NO MORE FREEZING

Freezing is the name given to a temporary and involuntary inability to move. When freezing occurs, your feet can feel like they are glued to the floor. You are basically stuck there standing. Attempts to move are useless or you may lose your balance trying. Freezing typically happens under predictable circumstances, but can also happen randomly. You may experience freezing episodes when crossing thresholds, entering or exiting elevators, or when turning corners. Unfortunately, freezing does not always respond to an increase or adjustment of medications; however, there are various techniques that can be used to reduce the duration and incidence of freezing episodes. This is where you have to establish your "personal trick". If you do not have a personal trick, you could be stuck in a position for quite some time or actually fall. Here are some tricks for you to consider.

Anti- Freezing Strategies
✓ Stop when freezing occurs. Do not attempt to move through it, as this often leads to loss of balance.
✓ Restart movement with a purposeful step (*See Poor Man's Hula*).

17

✓ Visualize stepping over an imaginary object.
✓ If doorways and elevators are a problem, try to look past the threshold focusing on where you want to go, versus the threshold itself.
✓ See what tricks work for you and practice these strategies. Having done this may decrease anxiety, lessening the "freezing effect."

TIP: Poor Man's Hula: When a freezing episode occurs the 1st thing to do is just stop. Then slowly shift your weight from side to side. I call it the "poor man's hula". The "hula" will prepare you to reinitiate moving. With freezing, you will typically have weight on both feet not freeing up either of your two legs. Now deliberately shift weight to one leg (hula) and purposefully pick up the opposite foot to reinitiate stepping. It may take a little practice, but this technique can be in your bag of tricks if freezing occurs. It works well to get in the habit of always performing this the same way each time by always shifting to one specific leg and always stepping with same opposite leg. The more you practice, the more effective this will be when you need it.

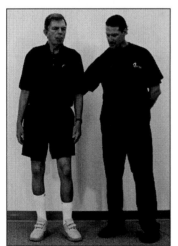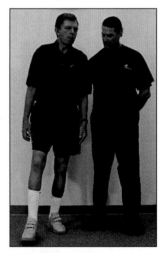

**Poor man's hula sequence used to off-load one leg
to free up the opposite leg to step with.**

FINDING YOUR PERSONAL TRICK (Anti-Freeze)

Freezing can sometimes be predictable, but other times it just happens without warning. Considering the presented strategies, it is important for you to establish a trick to get you out of trouble. Here is an example that may be helpful for you in finding your personal trick. There was a gentleman with PD who liked to work on his computer in his study which was away from other rooms in his home. When he needed to get up he would reach for a book shelf that was above his computer and pull himself into standing. Once he was standing, he was still leaning forward with his hands on the shelf when he became frozen. This consistently happened every time he tried this maneuver. He said that he has been stuck in this position for over an hour on many occasions. He tried to yell for his wife but the room was far away from the other areas in his home and he had some difficulty with projecting his voice, which is another typical symptom of PD.

Okay, so now we wanted to help this gentleman find his personal trick. The first issue was that his center of gravity was way in front of his base of support. So we had to fix that first. The first move was to perform the "posture" correction of tightening the buttocks and squeezing the shoulder blades together which will bringing his center of gravity back over the feet, his base of support. Now, we needed to get him moving by performing the poor man's hula, shifting weight side to side and initiating a first big step. Then, VIOLA! He was unfrozen. With just 3 minutes of practice, this gentleman was able to consistently get out this frozen state in less than 60 seconds! He perfected his personal trick!

TIP : One anti-falling technique taught to me by one of my patients with long-standing PD is to throw your arms up in the air if you find yourself falling. This type of movement could occur if you are going to fall forward due to forward posturing and the initiation of the fast shuffling gait. It brings your center of gravity back enough to right

19

yourself and stops the forward progression that most likely will lead to a fall. After regaining your balance, you can then use the other mentioned techniques to reinitiate walking.

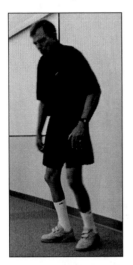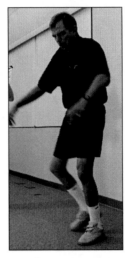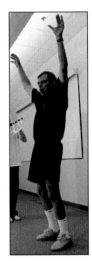

Anti-falling technique when your center of gravity is too far forward and you are shuffling your feet but they cannot catch up. Your center of gravity is "re-set" backwards by throwing your arms in the air.

TIP: One trick is to tie a small, colored ribbon on the end of your cane. When freezing occurs, focus on the bright colored ribbon and step past it to get out of your frozen state.

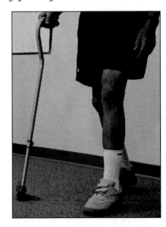

THE CURLY SHUFFLE (Walking Patterns of PD): Okay, you can hear each and every step you take and the front under-soles of your shoes are worn thin. Oftentimes you just get going and you can't stop. Your walking looks like this: shuffling feet, knees are bent the entire time, slumped posture, and no arm swing.

There are multiple gait abnormalities of lesser degree that show up first. One of the first notable gait changes is loss of arm swing on one side. Other abnormalities include a stiff-legged gait. This is basically when your knee stays stiff or you leave it or drag it behind you; however, if you were instructed to march you could flex and bring the leg forward. This is just another example of the need for conscious thought to move. With progressed PD, you can experience a "festinating gait" as mentioned above. This occurs when your walking speed uncontrollably quickens and can result in your breaking into a shuffling run in an effort to avoid falling.

VALUE OF EXTERNAL CUES FOR WALKING

Regardless of your progression of PD, there are simple strategies that you can use to improve your gait and decrease your risk for falling as your PD progresses. You have been hearing much about purposeful movement and as you can guess, walking is a great place to apply it. This goes back to the earlier statement about the "automatic pilot." Parkinson's Disease makes it (your automatic pilot) ineffective. In other words, prior to Parkinson's Disease, you did not have to think to move, but now, well, you do. What may be helpful is talking to your body. Actually tell the legs and arms when and how to move. You are simply cueing yourself. This technique brings your movement to a conscious level. The bottom line is that you can improve your gait and general movement with external cues. These can be either visual or auditory cues (or both) which will be some of the tricks you can use to improve mobility.

Another effective training tool is to use two broom sticks or two canes. Now you will perform a four-point walking pattern which goes like this: 1) stick, 2) opposite leg, 3) opposite stick, 4) opposite leg. It helps to talk to your body: "Arm, Leg, Arm, Leg". With each step, attempt to get your heel down first while your knee is fully extended. The "four-point gait" mimics the normal gait pattern. Advancing the pole with one arm simulates arm swing while advancing the opposite leg simulates a reciprocal gait pattern that promotes pelvic rotation. This technique is effective because it not only forces a normal walking pattern; but also forces purposeful movement which can train or retrain yourself to walk purposely.

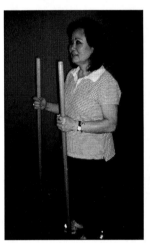 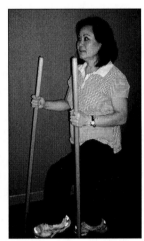 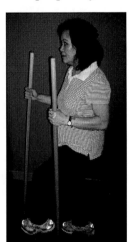

Four point gait

TIP : The "four-point gait" can be used and applied in many ways. If you have the balance and stability to walk without a walker but need some additional support for balance, you can use two canes or two walking/hiking sticks. Walking sticks are less "medical" looking and may be a good alternative. The "four point gait" can also be a strategy to combat "freezing." The purposeful movement brings your walking to a conscious level which can allow you to regain control of your movement. Some of my patients will pull out their "imaginary" canes and use the four-point walking pattern to unfreeze or to initiate walking. This is especially useful when having to get up in the middle of the night to use the restroom or during the wearing-off periods of your medication.

Walking Strategies

✓ Always initiate walking with a purposeful first step. It is often helpful to train yourself by taking the first step with the same leg each time.

✓ Start walking with a marching pattern. I call this the "British Soldier." After a few steps you can settle into a less obvious gait pattern. The marching pattern forces you to have a reciprocal arm swing as well as a good leg swing to decrease leg drag or the tendency to shuffle your feet.

✓ If shuffling of your feet occurs, purposefully attempt to get your heel down first with each step.

✓ If you continue to shuffle, STOP and restart with a purposeful step. Try not to work through the shuffle as it may lead to a fall.

✓ Allow your arms to swing freely. If you have one stiff arm, you can carry an object or swing a purse or bag with the stiff arm. The additional weight along with momentum can make it easier to engage the "stiff" arm in your walking pattern.

✓ Turn corners in a wide arc. Avoid crossing your feet over each other when turning.

Auditory Cues

Rhythmic auditory cues can improve your walking pattern. This can involve timed auditory cues such as clicks, beats, or taps given at specific intervals for learning a sequential activity. There have been multiple studies which have shown improved walking patterns using this technique. Some have involved practicing walking with a metronome to cue weight-shifting and stepping. Some folks hum or click a rhythmic pattern with their tongue to self cue their walking pattern. There was also a very recent study that showed tango dancing showed greater improvement in overall movement versus conventional exercises. This is probably due to the combination of teaching purposeful movements in combination with rhythmic auditory cues.

BED MOBILITY

With advancing PD symptoms, you may encounter some difficulty with what used to be easily performed daily tasks, including bed mobility. For some of you, moving from a lying position to sitting may be a very difficult task. There is a technique using simple mechanics and leverage that may allow you to perform this with greater ease.

Try this sequence below:

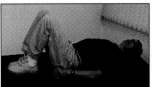 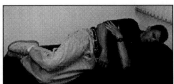 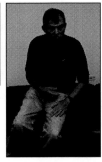

- Bend your knees until they are in a hook-lying position, in which your knees are bent and your feet are flat on the bed.

- Roll to side-lying and lower your legs off the bed. Your upper trunk will begin to pull up, allowing for you to have better leverage with you bottom arm.

- Push up to sitting.

ATTEMPTS TO STAND

Rising from a low surface or getting out of a car can be difficult, especially with progressed PD symptoms. You may find yourself making multiple attempts to stand up and often times you fall backwards into the car seat, chair, or bed. As in improving bed mobility, you can apply good mechanics and leverage to make this task easier.

The key is bending forward enough to get your center of gravity over your base of support. In other words, if your head and shoulders are behind your knees when you attempt to stand, you will push yourself backwards when you straighten out your knees. Ultimately you will fall back into the chair or seat. However, if you can bend forward at your hips to where your head and shoulders are in front of your knees, your body will rise because now your center of gravity is directly under your base of support. The cue I like to use is "get your nose past your toes." You may need to push or pull yourself to keep forward as you straighten out your legs. If you have someone to help you, the helper simply can lightly pull you forward from this flexed position while you do all of the work of managing to stand up. The helper doesn't need to lift you up but only keep you forward so you are at a mechanical advantage.

This technique is especially useful when trying to get up from a car seat. Car seats tend to be lower than an average chair (19" floor-to-seat). The bottom line is, the lower the surface you are rising from, the more you need to get yourself forward.

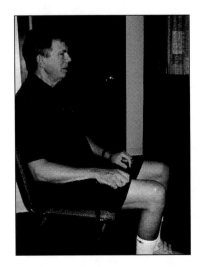

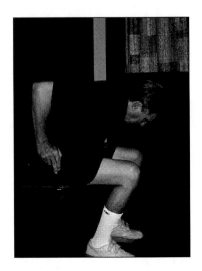

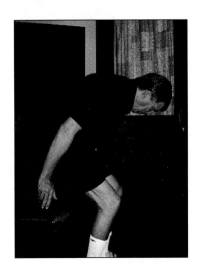

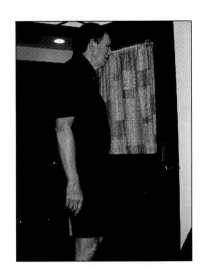

CHAPTER THREE

Assistive Devices

There is a spectrum of assistive devices available from minimal support to greater support. The timing of when and what device you will require is dependent on your specific needs. For the most part, persons with PD do not use assistive devices for the same reason that persons with other orthopedic issues may use the same device. For orthopedic reasons, most people use assistive devices to decrease weight-bearing on a particular leg. This could be due to pain or weakness from osteoarthritis in a hip or knee or some post-surgical condition resulting from a hip, knee, or ankle injury. With PD, it is more of an issue of balance versus the need to bear less weight on your legs. I will take you through a look at each device and present the profile and preferences for it.

Canes: A single point cane can be helpful for multiple reasons. It can provide minimal support for balance but can also be used to assist you in your walking. One way is that you purposefully step with the opposite foot to assist you in a more normal walking pattern that includes arm swing and pelvic rotation. Traditionally or with orthopedic injuries, you are instructed to use the cane on the opposite side of the injured leg. Many times with PD patients, I will recommend that the cane be used with the involved arm to promote arm swing and to re-engage that affected arm into your walking pattern. A single point can also be helpful in transitions through thresholds, and elevators. One tip mentioned earlier is to tie a small ribbon on the end of the cane to aid in placing the cane through the threshold first, then stepping towards or past the cane with the opposite foot. The whole time you are focusing on the ribbon or where you are stepping and not on the threshold itself. There are other types of canes that can give you more support if you need to bear more weight with your arms and less on one of your legs, such as small-base and large-base quad canes. I have not found these types of canes very useful at all, but rather clumsy to handle, so I rarely recommend quad canes for my patients with PD.

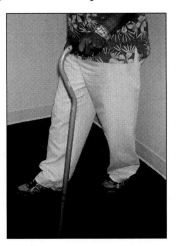 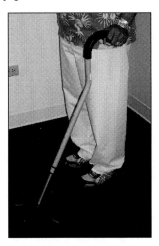

Walkers: There is a time and place for walkers, but I try to avoid them as long as possible because they can promote bad posture and an unnatural walking pattern. As we talked about earlier, there is a tendency toward "forward posturing" that places your center of gravity in front of your base of support. The walker almost forces this posture. Also, the walker completely takes away arm swing.

Arm swing plays a major role in assuring an efficient walking pattern by promoting pelvic rotation. Without pelvic rotation, we would have a more lateral quality to our gait (like Frankenstein) which is harder on our joints and not as efficient. Rarely do I recommend a pick-up walker for persons with PD. The most common recommendation is the front-wheeled rolling walker. This walker is easier to maneuver with PD because you do not have to pick it up. Even with a walker, you should try to walk with a step- through gait versus a step-to gait. Basically you try to step past the opposite foot instead of even with it. It is also important to try to step into the walker which means that you can't be bent over too much with the walker too far in front of you. If you are stepping into the walker with each step, you will be keeping a better posture and not contributing to the typical PD forward posturing or festinating gait. It may help you to tie a band or cloth across the front of the walker. This gives you a visual cue to step toward.

Another style of walker is the 4-wheeled walker. This style of walker typically comes with hand brakes and a fold-down seat. One concern with this type of walker is that for those with progressed PD where there is a higher likelihood of provoking a festinating gait, because this style of walker can have a tendency to get away from you. The last consideration with a walker is the height of the walker. The traditional way of measuring height of a walker (and a cane) is by standing tall with your arms relaxed down to your sides. You then raise or lower the walker until the handle is at or close to the bend of the wrist. You can then move it up or down one hole for comfort. The reason for this strategy is to allow for the most optimal leverage for the arms for bearing weight. Keep in mind, the traditional use of walkers is for orthopedic injuries in which you want the arms to do more work to lessen the burden on an injured leg. This is not typically true with PD. I tend to raise the walker much higher than the bend of the wrist to aid in posture. You will most likely be using the walker for balance and less for the purpose of decreasing weight-bearing by your legs.

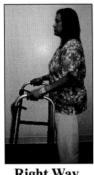 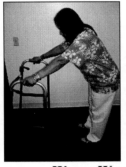 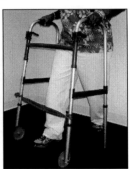

| Right Way | Wrong Way | External Cue for stepping |

Commercial Specialty Assistive Devices

Walking Aids with External Cues

There are many walking devices that are on the market to assist in overcoming some of the PD symptoms. Many of these devices were developed by people with PD. Below are samples of devices that you may want to further investigate. These devices are designed based on almost forcing purposeful movement to overcome "freezing." I do not endorse any one product but want to present some of the options that are available.

The NextStep® walking assistant unit becomes a part of your cane as it merely slides over the end.

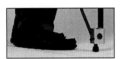 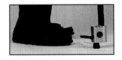 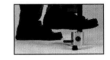

- When the cane comes into contact with the walking surface, the rod automatically lowers into place.

- With the cane pressed down on the walking surface, the rod becomes your obstacle to step over.

- With the cane in the right hand, step up and over the rod with your right foot.

- Now pull or drag your left foot forward until it is even with your right foot.

- As with any normal cane, next pick the cane up from the walking surface and bring it forward.

- As you place it down onto the walking surface, the rod automatically lowers into place.

- Now you are ready for your next step!

Parkinson Next Step, LLC © 2005-06
3227 Wellington Court, Raleigh, NC 27615
1-888-344-7837 • email: info@icanstep.com

U-Step Walking Stabilizer: It is not like pushing a walker. Instead, the U-Step surrounds you and moves with you. You will feel as stable as you would feel holding onto another person's arm.
The braking system is easy to use and puts you in complete control. The U-Step will not roll unless you are ready to walk. When you lightly squeeze a hand brake, the unit will roll with you. Once you release the hand brake, the unit will stop immediately. This feature is particularly helpful when standing up from a chair because the unit will not roll away from you.

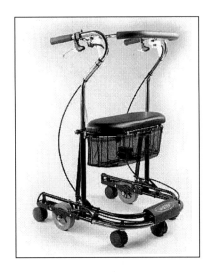

Laser Light: Laser Light™ helps prevent freezing. LaserLight™ is an exclusive optional feature of the U-Step. Simply press the red button on the handlebar and a bright red laser line is projected on the floor for you to step over. The laser offers a safe, obstacle-free visual cue that helps you break the "freezing episode," and walk normally with increased stride length.

This laser technology is also available with a cane. The laser is powered by two AA batteries, which are easy to replace and typically last at least six months.

In-Step Mobility Products Corp.

8027 N. Monticello Ave.

Skokie, IL 60076

1-800-558-7837

1-847-676-1275

walkers@ustep.com

www.ustep.com

CHAPTER FOUR

Falls: How To Minimize Them, How To Fall, And What To Do Once You Are On The Floor.

I wish that I could tell you that you will never fall, but the truth is that at some point as your PD progresses it is likely to happen. Because of this, it is important to know what you can do to minimize falls, how to fall, and what to do once you are on the floor. Research shows that falls are the leading cause of unintentional injury at home among Americans 65 and older. Persons with PD have a much higher likelihood for falling than the general population. Despite the statistics, many times falls can be prevented by understanding the different balance factors. You can either change or compensate for both the intrinsic and extrinsic factors that lead to falls. There were many intrinsic factors presented in chapter one, especially as it relates to posture. In this chapter we will explore the other intrinsic balance factors as well as discuss how to better fall-proof your environment (extrinsic factors).

PREVENTION

Intrinsic factors/risk for falling: Balance factors can be broken down into two categories. The first includes intrinsic factors which relate to your physical capabilities and characteristics and the second group, the extrinsic factors, relate to your environment or anything outside of your body. The three physical balance systems are vision, somatosensory/proprioception, and the vestibular system.

Vision: Age-related changes in vision can decrease the ability to accurately perceive changes in surface conditions or the presence of hazards in the environment. The increasing prevalence of eye diseases such as cataracts, glaucoma, and macular degeneration among older adults has also been associated with increasing fall rates. Regular eye exams and check-ups can decrease risk for falls by minimizing visual deficits allowing for better anticipation of changes in surfaces and in perception environmental hazards such as negotiating curbs, stairs, and uneven terrain.

Somatosensory/proprioception: The somatosensory system provides information about the spatial relationship of the body to the support surface. It is basically the ability to feel the surface you are on whether it is the firm surface of wood floors or the soft surface of a padded carpet. In the absence or decline in vision, the somatosensory system becomes the primary source of sensory information that provides balance as well as the capacity to move around in dark areas.

Vestibular system: The final balance system is the vestibular system. This is the system that is housed in the inner ear and is activated when one moves his head. The vestibular system becomes very important when the other two systems are impaired. Examples include walking on uneven terrain which disrupts the somatosensory system or the ability to feel in conjunction with really crowded areas or darker areas that can distort vision. The vestibular system is trainable and can be taught to better compensate for visual and/or sensory deficits.

Other intrinsic factors include posture changes and neurological conditions/diseases such as strokes and Parkinson's Disease.

Posture/osteoporosis: Good posture is critical to good balance and refers to the body's alignment. With age, some people can develop a kyphotic posture, which is a hump in the upper back. This posture causes a forward head and a hyperextension of the neck to be able to scan the environment in front versus looking at the ground. This postural change moves the center of gravity, making the person more susceptible to falling backwards when walking up a ramp or reaching overhead or falling forward when walking down a ramp.

Even though one may not have control over certain intrinsic factors such as macular degeneration, risks for falls can greatly be decreased by knowledge of your physical limitations and at-risk situations as well as training your body to compensate for impairments in one or more of the balance systems.

Extrinsic factors/risk for falling

In addition to the intrinsic factors, extrinsic factors can affect your risk for falls. The two primary external risk factors are medications and the physical environment.

Medications: If you are taking four or more prescription medications, you are at higher risk for falls. Certain medications have side effects that can contribute to that risk; the interactions of some drugs and supplements which can cause adverse effects leading to falls. Certain classes of prescription medication are associated with higher fall risk than others. These include sedatives/ hypnotics, antidepressants, and psychotropic medications. It is highly recommended that you keep a consolidated drug list to share with your primary care physician or any specialist so that they are aware of what you are taking before prescribing any new medication. If you are uncertain, it is best to put all of the supplements and prescription medications in a bag and take them to your primary care physician or pharmacist.

Environment: The second external factor that can have direct impact on your fall risk is your physical environment itself. Many hazards in your home may include floor rugs that are not secured down, exposed electrical or appliance cords, poor lighting, lack of grab bars in the restroom, clutter, too-soft plush carpet, absence of night lights, cabinets too high, furniture too low, awkward thresholds into different rooms, etc.

Below are some simple home safety strategies:

a. Lighting: Make sure corridors are well lighted.

b. Nightlights: Use of night-lights can aid in better vision in the middle of the night.

c. Throw rugs: either remove or secure rugs down with 2-way carpet tape.

d. Clutter: Reduce clutter that interferes with clear walking paths.

e. Low-toilets: Use raised commode seat and/or install grab bars.

f. Cabinets: Store items in lower areas or redesign cabinets to be lower or accessible without need of a stepstool.

g. Low seats: Replace furniture with pieces that have a higher seat-to-floor height or have one chair that has a seat-to-floor height that you can rise from without difficulty.

h. Heavily padded plush carpet: This type of carpet disrupts proprioception or your ability to feel, placing you at greater risk for falls. Replace with low-pile carpet, tile, or wood.

See our appendix for a Home Assessment Checklist

Fall Prevention strategies

In addition to checking out your medications and improving the safety of your physical environment, exercise can greatly reduce your risk for falls. Studies show that older adults with greater quadricep strength (knee extensor muscle) show a much reduced risk for falls than older adults with lesser strength in the same muscle groups. General physical condition can affect your risk for falls. It is very common for individuals to experience loss of balance and/ or falls following prolonged bed-rest or hospitalization. In these circumstances, not only do the muscles experience weakness and possibly atrophy, but the vestibular system is not as efficient when not challenged or stressed at all due to inactivity.

Balance is a skill that can be restored or improved via specific exercises and activity. Simple measures, such as having a physician or pharmacist review prescription medications and assessing your environment, also can aid greatly in reducing the overall risk for falls.

How to fall and what do I do once I get there (on the floor)

Falling

You don't ever plan on falling; however, with some training you can possibly minimize serious injury with practicing falls. When possible, you want to try to protect your head and to break your fall with your hands in a cupped position and then roll off to one side on your buttocks or shoulder. Direct impact to the hip or shoulder can cause fractures and/or dislocations. If you are falling backward, lean your head forward and try to hit with your buttocks first. Leaning forward may lessen the impact and will have a better likelihood of avoiding hitting your head. Contact with the buttocks first versus falling to your side directly on your hip can also lessen the chance of a hip fracture, which is common with falls.

Getting up from the floor

Now you are on the floor, if you are unsure about any serious injury such as a hip, shoulder, or spine fracture, it is best to lie flat and call for help. If you are okay then you can follow the following sequence to get up:

1) Roll to your side curled up into "fetal position."

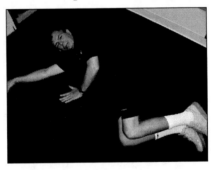

2) Push up on your bottom arm so that you are resting on your elbow.

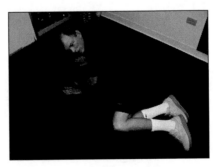

3) Roll to an all-four position.

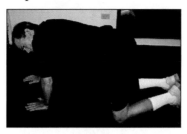

4) Walk your hands up your thigh until you are in "tall kneeling" position or if a chair, couch or bed is close, crawl or walk on all fours until you reach the chair and use you arms to assist you into tall kneeling.

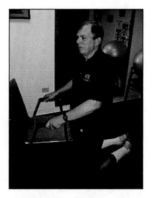

5) Shift your weight to one side and place your strongest foot forward to a "half kneeling" position.

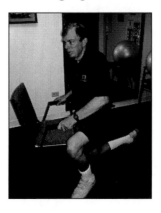

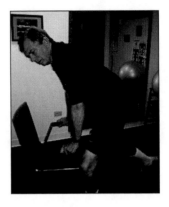

6) Lean forward, push off your strong leg until both feet are underneath you.

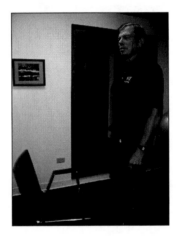

7) Squeeze your buttocks tight and pinch your shoulder blades together and extend your self to upright standing.

CHAPTER FIVE

Adaptive Devices For Easier Daily Living

Arlene Ono OT

The physical symptoms of PD can make daily living activities challenging. Tremors, rigidity, bradykinesia, and postural instability affect tasks in various ways. We'll look at some common problems and adaptive devices and strategies that may be helpful.

Grooming: An electric razor increases safety and ease of shaving. Larger handle hairbrushes and toothbrushes are easier to grip. If you are having difficulty controlling fine movements, an electric toothbrush can help with thoroughly brushing your teeth. Also, if you tend to lose your balance backwards, it may be safer to sit while you do your grooming routine.

Upper extremity (UE) Dressing: If you have a problem with your posture or balance, you may find it easier to sit to put on a shirt or sweater. If one arm is more rigid or has more tremors than the other, it is usually easier to dress that side first. Looser fitting clothing, larger buttons, and Velcro fasteners are some helpful options. If you are having difficulty removing a blouse or shirt, grabbing the

41

shirt from behind the neck and pulling it over your head may make it easier. Many times, buttoning is difficult for someone with PD. A device which many people find helpful is a button aid.

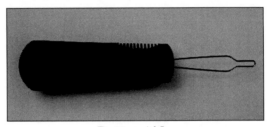

Button Aide

Lower extremity (LE) Dressing: It is usually safer and easier to put your feet into shorts or pants either while leaning against a wall, or sitting. If you have difficulty reaching down to your feet, you may benefit from using a reacher or dressing stick to get the pant legs over your feet. There are various styles of sock aids which may help to get your feet into the socks. A long-handled shoe horn is helpful for putting on shoes. Velcro closures make fastening shoes easier and elastic shoelaces convert a laced shoe into a slip-on shoe.

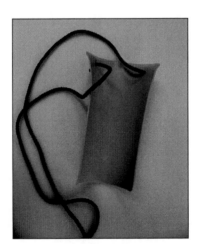

Sock Aide

Bathing: Grab bars in the tub or shower can help you enter and exit safely. A rubber mat or non-skid decals on the tub or shower floor help to prevent slips and falls. Sitting on a bath bench to bathe also helps if you have problems with your balance and have difficulty reaching your feet. Soap on a rope keeps soap within reach and prevents you from dropping it. Liquid soap and shampoo in a pump bottles may also be easier to manage. There are bath brushes and sponges that can help with reaching your back and feet to wash.

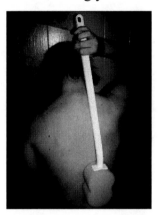

Bath reacher sponge

Eating: Tremors and rigidity can interfere with eating. Some people find weighted utensils help to control the tremors. Also, angled utensils make scooping and inserting food into the mouth easier and neater. In addition, a plate guard creates a ledge on a plate which food can be scooped against and prevents spillage. If you are having difficulty cutting up food, you may want to use a rocker knife.

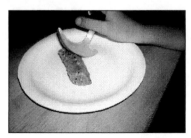
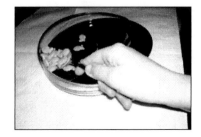

Writing: Like weighted utensils for eating, weighted writing instruments may help reduce the effects of tremors on writing legibility. Wider grip pens and pencils are usually easier to use than standard-sized instruments. Micrographia, or the tendency to write smaller and smaller, is a common symptom of PD. Oftentimes, you may be able to start off writing legibly, and as you continue on in a sentence or paragraph, the writing becomes progressively smaller. One strategy that may be helpful is to pause when your writing begins to get smaller, consciously "think big," then start writing again.

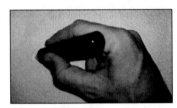

Meal Preparation: It is helpful to organize your kitchen so that frequently used items are placed within reach (as close to waist height as possible). A reacher can help you to pick up objects from the floor or from a high shelf. A rubberized shelf liner or a wet dishcloth placed under bowls, pans and cutting boards will stabilize them while you prepare food.

You will find that various styles of cutting boards with raised edges and nails to keep food from falling off the board will stabilize food while you are slicing or chopping it. If you have difficulty opening cans, an electric can opener is helpful. Different types of jar openers my also be useful to you.

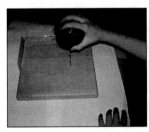 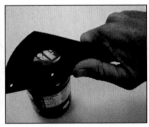 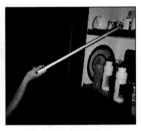

Adapted Cutting Board   **Jar Opener**   **Reacher**

CHAPTER SIX

Role And Importance Of Exercise

Focus on posture and purposeful movement is the key to an effective exercise program with PD. The postural muscles are important to maintaining range of motion in the shoulders for activities of daily living. They control balance and gait by keeping your center gravity over your base of support (your feet), while assisting you in fatigue. The main antigravity and postural muscles are your scapular muscles/upper back, back/hip extensors and your quadriceps. The stronger your postural muscles are, the better equipped you will be to battle "forward posturing," the tendency toward pulling or stooping forward. There are many ways to exercise these key muscle groups. In this book we will go over different routines that will give you exercise options at home or in a community fitness setting. Routines will be presented for you to simply follow along. The routines will be divided into 3 levels. You can choose the level that best fits your mobility profile.

PD Exercise Research

Recent studies have shown that exercise can have beneficial effects in patients with Parkinson's Disease. One study looked at treadmill exercise and its effects in animal models with and without a loss of cells similar to those a PD sufferer typically loses. Given the importance of dopamine in Parkinson's Disease, the researchers looked at changes in dopamine levels. They found that exercise had an effect on the dopamine level of the subjects with cell loss but did little to alter the levels in those with normal cell readings. A study by Viliani, Pasquetti, Magnolfi et al aimed to evaluate whether motor training could improve the straightening-up movements in patients with Parkinson's Disease. Consequently, they found that such training could enhance the capacity of the patients to change the body's position. The results showed statistically significant differences in all the motor parameters that were evaluated (supine to sitting and sitting to supine, supine rolling, standing from a chair). Researchers concluded that physical training can be effective in improving motor performance related to changes in position, clearly affecting the simple daily activities of the patients.

Many other studies have been done and many are currently underway. More research is needed to fully understand the effects of exercise on Parkinson's Disease and the underlying reasons for the effects.

Your Body's Response

We are addressing the physiological effects of strength training to give you a better understanding of how your body will react to an exercise program you design for yourself. Understanding the cause and effects will help you to better design and modify your exercise program to meet your needs and goals. It is important to note that PD works on a particular area in your brain but does not directly work on your muscles, so your muscles still can have the ability to maintain strength and flexibility if you train them. A study by Scandalis, Bosak, Berliner et al showed that patients with mild-to-moderate Parkinson's disease can obtain increases in performance or strength similar to that of normal adults of the same age in a resistance training program. Resistance training can produce functional improvements in gait and may, therefore, be useful as part of a physical rehabilitation and/or health maintenance program for people with Parkinson's Disease.

The human body has a remarkable ability to adapt to the stresses placed on it. When the muscle fibers and the anaerobic energy system are stressed by weightlifting or resistive training, they adapt. With appropriate stress on these systems, rest, and recuperation, the muscle will become stronger as a positive adaptation to the stress put on it.

Initial gains in strength are most likely due to both effects on the muscles and the nervous system. The nervous system stimulates and controls the muscles. During the initial training phase, the nervous system basically learns the skill of the movements (exercises) and learns how to efficiently recruit the muscle fibers to develop the best coordination for those desired motions.

BASIC TRAINING PRINCIPLES AND CONSIDERATIONS

Progressive Resistive Exercise (PRE)

As a muscle adapts to applied stresses, resistance must gradually be increased for further positive changes to occur, thus the term progressive resistive exercise. Large increases in resistance should be avoided; if the stress is too great, you could injure your muscle or tendons. If your increase in resistance results in poor technique, then it is too much weight. One guide that you can use is to make sure that the last 2-3 repetitions are at least somewhat challenging. If repetitions 8,9,10 are as easy as repetitions 1,2,3 you may want to challenge yourself more.

Sets and Repetitions

With use of the appropriate training load, the number of sets and repetitions governs the goal and outcome of the exercise program. Sets and repetitions can be set up for muscular endurance, muscular strength, and muscular power routines. Core muscles such as the scapular and pelvic girdle musculature are best trained via a muscular endurance routine since they are chiefly endurance and postural muscles. Since keeping or achieving a more upright posture is key, it is best to train your muscles for muscular endurance.

Muscular Endurance Routine
is 8-20 reps/ 3-5 sets with Low to Medium training load

General recommendations

Consult closely with your doctor, physical therapist or healthcare professional before designing and beginning your exercise program.

General recommendations for getting started include:
✓ Aim for at least 15 minutes of exercise every day.
✓ Make sure to include a thorough stretching program that targets each joint and muscle group.
✓ Spend a few minutes warming up and cooling down. This could include marching in place or stretching.
✓ Start with the easiest exercises first. Slowly introduce the more difficult exercises as your level of fitness increases.
✓ Try to perform each movement to the best of your ability.
✓ If you suffer from fatigue, try exercising first thing in the morning.

Safety suggestions

If you are at risk of falling,

General Safety Suggestions Include:

✓ Perform your exercises sitting down (or)

✓ Hold onto a chair when performing standing exercises.

✓ Don't perform floor exercises if you can't get up by yourself.

✓ Only exercise when other people are at home who can help if necessary.

✓ Exercise with others.

✓ Ask for assistance from a family member or friend.

Walking for fitness

Walking is excellent for overall fitness.

Suggestions Include:

✓ Choose flat, obstacle-free terrain.

✓ Taking larger strides may help you keep better balanced.

✓ Focus on lifting each foot and placing it down heel first.

✓ Count each step – this can help to make a smoother, more rhythmic walking style.

✓ Move your arms as you walk, if possible.

✓ If walking isn't practical or possible, explore other options such as stationary bicycling.

EXERCISE LEVELS & PROFILES

If you made it this far, you are now ready to learn about and perform the exercises that will assist you in staving off some of the physical symptoms of PD. We will go over different routines that will give you exercise options at home regardless of your level of mobility. The routines will be divided into 3 levels/profiles. You will choose the level that best fits your mobility profile that is presented below.

LEVEL ONE: Moderate to severe symptomatic (wheelchair or walking with walker with assistance)

LEVEL TWO: Moderate symptomatic (impaired balance requires assistive device.)

LEVEL THREE: Mildly symptomatic (standing balance good, no assistive device)

The exercises presented are not all inclusive but rather a selection of exercises that are specific to combat the forward/flexed posturing of PD. Maintaining strength and muscular endurance in your postural muscles or anti-gravity muscles is essential. The muscle groups that we will focus on are your scapular or upper back muscles, hip extensors, back extensors, and knee extensors. You will find that the programs presented do not focus on your anterior muscles such as your chest, bicep, etc. It is okay to exercise these muscles as well, as long as you prioritize the postural muscles.

CHAPTER SEVEN

Level One Exercises

LEVEL ONE: Moderate to severe symptomatic (wheelchair or walking with walker with assistance)

This group of exercises is good for anyone because it does not require balance in stance. These exercises are especially appropriate for you if you are wheelchair bound or are using assistive devices that require bilateral upper extremity support such as a walker. The exercises in this category are primarily performed while sitting or lying down. We recommend that you start out with 1 set of 10 repetitions for each exercise and build up to performing 2-3 sets of 10, as you can tolerate it. We suggest that you also break up the exercises into different days so that you are not performing such a large volume of exercises at one time. One suggestion is to perform the sitting exercise on opposite days of the mat exercises. A good schedule may involve performing the sitting group on Monday, Wednesday, Friday and the mat exercise group on Tuesday and Thursday. The following week, you can reverse the days. We also recommend that you limit your time to spending 20-30 minutes maximum per exercise session. It is much better to get into the habit of exercising daily for 15-20 minutes than to skip days and then do too much to make up for missing days. If you do not get through all of the exercises in the list, just pick up where you left off on the next day you perform that group (sitting or mat) of exercises.

SUGGESTED EXERCISE LIST

Sitting exercise routine.

1) Static wall sitting

2) Wall sitting arm raise

3) Wall sitting arm diagonals

4) Wall sitting alternative leg lifts

5) Wall sitting alternate arm/leg lifts

6) Wood chop

Mat exercise routine

1) Bridges

2) Lower trunk rotation

3) Alternating leg lifts

4) Alternating arm/leg lifts

SITTING WALL EXERCISES

The sitting wall exercises are appropriate for you if you are wheelchair bound or use assistive devices that require bilateral upper extremity support, such as a walker.

Wall sitting

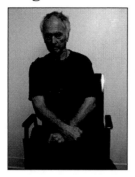 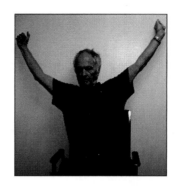

Beginning

EXERCISE POSITION: Sit with buttocks completely at back of a chair with shoulders and head against a wall with arms up and hold posture for 30 seconds.

PURPOSE: The emphasis is on promoting an erect posture. The contact with the wall gives the postural muscles feedback and a guide. The tendency is for PD symptoms to pull you forward. Many of you may feel like someone is behind you pushing you forward as your muscles may no longer hold you up straight. If you can retrain your muscles to maintain a more erect posture, your skeletal system will be more mechanically stacked actually requiring less energy to maintain an upright posture.

Wall sitting arm raise

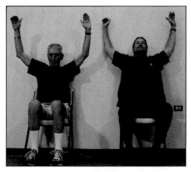

Beginning

START POSITION: Sit with buttocks all the way back in your chair with shoulders and head against a wall. Bring up your arms to the sides so that your elbow is same level as your shoulder with your elbow bent to 90 degrees. Maintain as much contact of your arms with the wall as possible.

ACTION/FINISH POSITION: Squeeze your shoulder blades together and maintain full contact with the wall as you slowly raise your arms overhead until your arms are completely straight. Hold this position for 10 seconds and slowly return to the start position.

PURPOSE: To stimulate and work the postural muscles as you move your arms. This exercise also promotes stability of your scapular muscles which will assist in maintaining functional strength and range of motion in your arms for activities of daily living.

Wall sitting alternating leg lifts

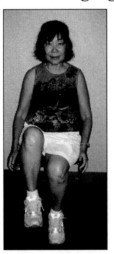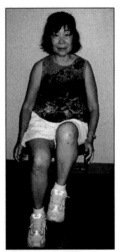

START POSITION: Sit with buttocks as far back in chair as possible with shoulders and head against a wall.

ACTION/FINISH POSITION: While maintaining contact with the wall, *purposely* shift your weight to the right leg and lift the opposite leg (left) like you are marching. Return to the start position and perform to the opposite side and repeat by alternating the leg lift and weight shift.

PURPOSE: To stimulate and work the postural muscles as you weight shift to move your legs. This exercise promotes good posture while you move dynamically and trains you in "anti-freezing techniques" by consciously, purposely engaging in controlled movement.

Wall sitting alternating arm- leg lifts

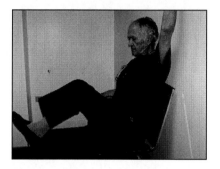 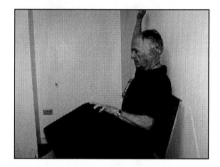

START POSITION: Sit with buttocks as far back in chair as possible with shoulders and head against a wall.

ACTION/FINISH POSITION: While maintaining contact with the wall, *purposely* shift your weight to the right leg and lift the opposite leg (left) while you simultaneously raise your right opposite arm (right). Return to the start position and perform to the opposite side and repeat by lifting your opposite arm/leg.

PURPOSE: To stimulate and work the postural muscles as you weight shift which off loads the opposite leg. This exercise promotes good posture while you move dynamically and trains you in "anti-freezing techniques" by consciously, purposely engaging in controlled movement.

Wall Sitting Arm Diagonals

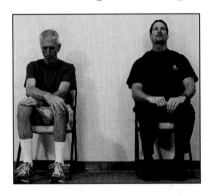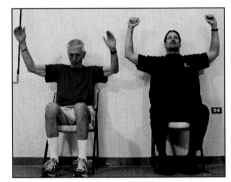

START POSITION: Sit with buttocks as far back as possible in chair with shoulders and head against a wall with each hand over the opposite hip.

ACTION/FINISH POSITION: Maintaining contact with the wall during the exercise. Squeeze your shoulder blades together while lifting your arms simultaneously in a diagonal position until your arms are extended and straightened out overhead.

PURPOSE: To stimulate and work the postural muscles as you move your arms. This exercise also promotes stability of your scapular muscles which will assist in maintaining functional strength and range of motion in your arms for activities of daily living.

Wood chop

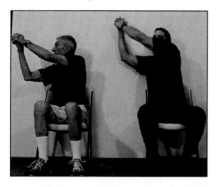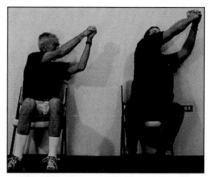

START POSITION: Sit with buttocks as far back as possible in chair with shoulders and head against wall. Grasp hands and place on the sides of one knee.

ACTION/FINISH POSITION: Lift your arms from the outside of your knee up towards and over the opposite shoulder while rotating your upper trunk in the direction your hands are moving. Return your hands back to the middle of your lap and repeat motion to other side.

PURPOSE: To stimulate and work trunk rotation which will assist in maintaining functional strength and range of motion in your shoulders and trunk for activities of daily living.

MAT EXERCISES

The mat exercises do not require very much balance and are appropriate for everyone as long as you can achieve the required positions. The positions that may be the most difficult to achieve are the exercises requiring you to lie on your stomach. The focus of mat exercises are the same as the wall exercises, which is to encourage purposeful movement and to strengthen the postural muscles to better combat the forward posturing and other related PD symptoms. All exercises in this set are done in a supine position, lying on one's back.

Bridges full arm contact

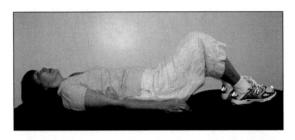

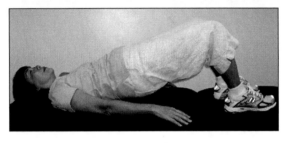

START POSITION: Lie down on your back with your arms extended by your side. Bend both of your knees so that your feet are flat on the mat or bed.

ACTION/FINISH POSITION: Hold your stomach tight as you squeeze your buttocks muscles and lift your buttocks as high off the mat or bed as possible. Hold the bridge position for 5 seconds and return to the start position.

PURPOSE: This exercise focuses on the postural muscles for hip and back extension. Your hip and back extensors will aid you in maintaining the strength and motion for a more upright posture.

Alternate arm positions for bridges (More challenging)

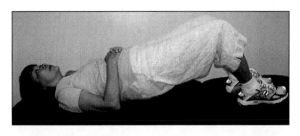

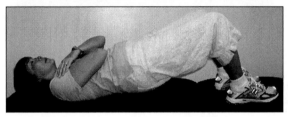

START POSITION: Lie down on your back with your elbows in contact with the bed or mat and arms resting on stomach or with arms crossed on chest. These alternate arm positions lessen the contact of the upper extremities making the exercise more challenging. Bend both of your knees so that your feet are flat on the mat or bed.

ACTION/FINISH POSITION: Hold your stomach tight as you squeeze your buttocks muscles and lift your buttocks as high off the mat or bed as possible. Hold the bridge position for 5 seconds and return to the start position.

PURPOSE: This exercise focuses on the postural muscles for hip and back extension. Your hip and back extensors will aid in maintaining the strength and motion for a more upright posture.

Lower trunk rotation (wind shield washers):

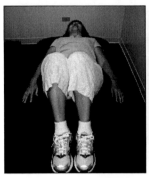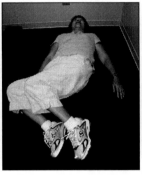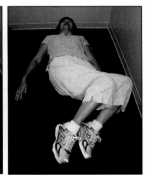

START POSITION: Lie down on your back with your arms extended by your side. Bend both of your knees so that your feet are flat on the mat or bed.

ACTION/FINISH POSITION: Maintain your shoulders in contact with the bed during the entire exercise. While keeping your knees and feet together, roll your knees as far to the right as possible (You will feel a stretch on the opposite side). Hold for 3 seconds and then roll your knees as far as possible to the left side. Return to starting position and then repeat for the desired amount of repetitions.

PURPOSE: This exercise focuses on trunk rotation. Flexibility in your trunk or pelvic rotation is essential for maintaining an efficient walking pattern as well as general mobility, such as getting in and out of a car or out of bed.

Alternating Leg Lifts

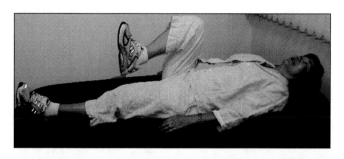

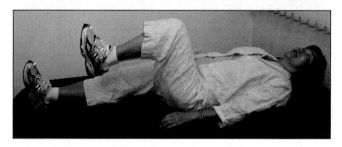

Beginning

START POSITION: Lie flat with arms down to side and legs extended.

ACTION/FINISH POSITION: While maintaining contact with the mat or bed, *purposely* shift your weight to the right leg and lift the opposite leg (left) like you are marching lying down. Return to starting position and perform to opposite side and repeat by alternately lifting your legs.

PURPOSE: To stimulate and work the postural muscles as you shift weight to off load the opposite leg. This exercise promotes good posture while you move dynamically and trains you in "anti-freezing techniques" by consciously, purposely engaging in controlled movement.

Alternating arm-leg lifts

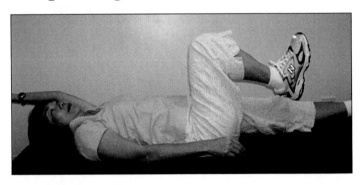

START POSITION: Lie flat with arms down at sides and legs extended.

ACTION/FINISH POSITION: While maintaining contact with the mat or bed, *purposely* shift your weight to the right leg and lift the opposite leg (left) as though you are marching lying down while concurrently raising your opposite arm over your head. Return to starting position and perform to the opposite side and repeat by alternately lifting your arm with opposite leg.

PURPOSE: To stimulate and work the postural muscles as you weight shift to off load the opposite leg. This exercise promotes a more normal gait with arm swing and trains you in "anti-freezing techniques" by consciously, purposely engaging in controlled movement.

CHAPTER EIGHT

Level Two Exercises

LEVEL TWO: Moderate symptomatic (impaired balance requires assistive device.)

This group of exercises is good for those of you with minimal to moderate impaired balance. These exercises may also require more complex movements, involving multiple limbs that require greater coordination than simpler exercises. If you have a history of falling and/or use an assistive device that requires just one hand (such as a cane), you may find these exercises appropriate. You may also modify the more advanced leg and balance exercises by using some support of your arms. If your balance is impaired to a level that does not allow for you to safely perform exercises in stance, please proceed to the sitting and mat exercises (Level One).

We recommend you start out with 1 set of 10 repetitions for each exercise and build up to performing 2-3 sets of 10 as you can tolerate it. We suggest that you also break up the exercises into different days so that you are not performing such a large volume of exercises at one time. One suggestion is to perform the sitting exercise on opposite days of the mat exercises. A good schedule would be to perform the sitting group on Monday, Wednesday, Friday and the mat exercise group on Tuesday and Thursday. The following week, you can then reverse the days. I also recommend that you limit your time to spending 20-30 minutes maximum per exercise session. It is much better to get into the habit of exercising daily for 15-20 minutes than to skip days then do too much to make up for missing days. If you do not get through all of the exercises in the list, just pick up where you left off the next day you perform that group (sitting or mat) of exercises.

SUGGESTED EXERCISE LIST:
Modified Standing Exercise routine.
1) Static wall standing with chair

2) Wall standing arm raise

3) Wall standing arm diagonals

4) Wall squats with chair

Mat exercise routine
1) Bridges

2) Lower Trunk Rotation

3) Supermans

4) Airplanes

STANDING WALL EXERCISES
The standing exercises in this category will require the ability for general balance with or without the need for upper extremity support. If your balance is impaired to the level that does not allow you to safely perform the standing exercises, please proceed to sitting and mat exercises.

Static Wall Standing

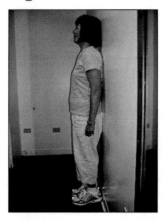

EXERCISE POSITION: Stand with heels, buttocks, shoulders and head against wall and hold this posture for 30 seconds.

PURPOSE: The emphasis is on promoting erect posture. The contact with the wall gives the postural muscles feedback and a guide. The tendency is to let the PD symptoms pull you forward. Many of you may feel like someone is behind you pushing you forward as your muscles may not be used to holding you up straight. If you can retrain your muscles to maintain a more erect posture, your skeletal system will be more mechanically stacked, actually requiring less energy to maintain an upright position.

EXERCISE MODIFICATION FOR DECREASED BALANCE: You can also perform the above exercise with a walker or tall back chair turned around and in front of you. Try to minimize the weight-bearing by your arms, but you will have the comfort of the support for safety.

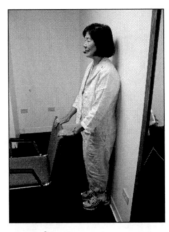

Wall standing arm raise

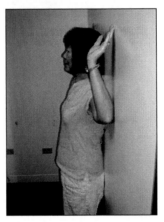

START POSITION: Stand with heels, buttocks, shoulders and head against wall. Bring your arms up so that your elbows, bent at 90 degrees, are at the same level as your shoulders. Maintain as much contact of your arms with the wall as possible.

ACTION/FINISH POSITION: Squeeze your shoulder blades together and maintain full contact with the wall as you slowly raise your arms overhead until your arms are completely straight. Hold this position for 10 seconds and slowly return back to the start position.

PURPOSE: To stimulate and work the postural muscles as you move your arms. This exercise also promotes stability of your scapular muscles which will assist in maintaining functional strength and range of motion in your arms for activities of daily living.

Wall standing alt leg lift

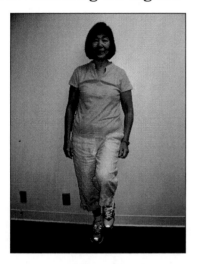 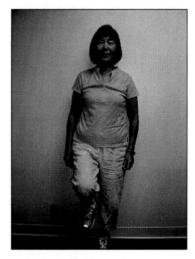

START POSITION: Stand with heels, buttocks, shoulders and head against the wall.

ACTION/FINISH POSITION: While maintaining contact with the wall, purposely shift your weight to the right leg and lift the left leg. Return to start position and perform in the opposite direction and repeat by alternately lifting your legs.

PURPOSE: To stimulate and work the postural muscles as you shift weight to off-load your opposite leg. This exercise promotes good posture while you move dynamically and trains you in "anti-freezing techniques" by consciously, purposely engaging in controlled movement.

EXERCISE MODIFICATION FOR DECREASED BALANCE:
You can also perform the above exercise with a walker or tall back chair turned around and to the side of you. Try to minimize the weight-bearing by your arms, but you have the comfort of the support for safety.

Wall Standing Diagonals

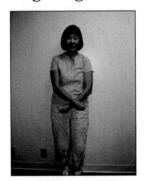 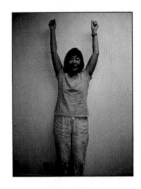

Intermediate

START POSITION: Stand with heels, buttocks, shoulders and head against the wall with each hand over the opposite hip.

ACTION/FINISH POSITION: Maintain contact with the wall during the exercise. Squeeze your shoulder blades together while lifting your arms simultaneously in a diagonal position until your arms are extended and straightened.

PURPOSE: To stimulate and work the postural muscles as you move your arms. This exercise also promotes stability of your scapular muscles which will assist in maintaining functional strength and range of motion in your arms for activities of daily living.

Wall standing squats

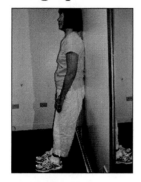 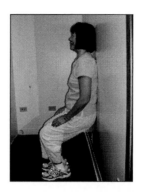

START POSITION: Stand with heels approximately 18 inches away from the wall with your buttocks, shoulders and head against the wall.

ACTION/FINISH POSITION: Maintain your buttock, shoulders, and head in contact with the wall while you slide down the wall. The bottom of the squat position will be dictated by your strength, but you should not squat deeper than 90 degrees at the hip, which occurs when your hip and knees are at the same level. The deeper the squat, the greater strength is required. One modification, in which you place your feet further away from the wall, decreases weight-bearing and makes the exercise easier.

PURPOSE: To stimulate and work the postural muscles, in particular the hip extensors (gluteals) and knee extensors (quadriceps).

MAT EXERCISES

The mat exercises do not require very much balance and are appropriate for everyone as long as you can achieve the required positions. The positions that may be the most difficult to achieve are the exercises during which you lie on your stomach. The focus of mat exercises are the same as the wall exercises, which is to encourage purposeful movement and to strengthen the postural muscles to better combat the forward posturing and other related PD symptoms. All exercises in this set are performed from the supine position, lying on the back.

Bridges

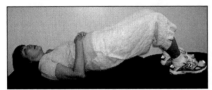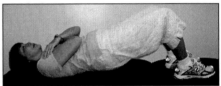

START POSITION: Lie down on your back with your elbows in contact with the bed or mat and arms resting on stomach or with arms crossed on chest. These alternate arm positions lessen the contact of the upper extremities, making the exercise more challenging. Bend both of your knees so that your feet are flat on the mat or bed.

ACTION/FINISH POSITION: Hold your stomach tight as you squeeze your buttocks muscles and lift your buttocks as high off the mat or bed as possible. Hold the bridge position for 5 seconds and return to starting position.

PURPOSE: This exercise focuses on the postural muscles for hip and back extension. Your hip and back extensors will aid you in maintaining the strength and motion for a more upright posture.

Lower trunk rotation (wind shield washers):

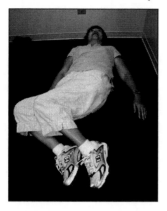 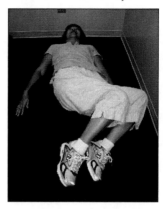

Beginning

START POSITION: Lie down on your back with your arms extended at your sides. Bend both of your knees so that your feet are flat on the mat or bed.

ACTION/FINISH POSITION: Maintain your shoulders in contact with the bed during the entire exercise. While keeping your knees and feet together, roll your knees as far to the right as possible (You will feel a stretch on the opposite side). Hold for 3 seconds and then roll your knees as far as possible to the left side. Return to starting position and then repeat for the desired amount of repetitions.

PURPOSE: This exercise focuses on trunk rotation. Flexibility in your trunk or pelvic rotation is essential for maintaining an efficient walking pattern as well as general mobility, such as getting in and out of a car or out of bed.

Supermans

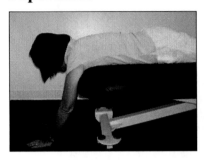 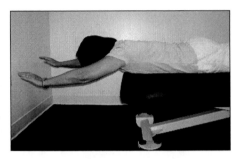

START POSITION: Lie flat on your stomach with your arms hanging down over the edge of your mat or bed.

ACTION/FINISH POSITION: Lift your arms straight up in front of you as high as you can as if you are flying like superman. Hold this position for 5 seconds and repeat to complete the desired amount of repetitions. Keep your head and neck neutral with your gaze straight down. Do not gaze forward, because this will hyper-extend your neck.

PURPOSE: To stimulate the postural muscles in your upper back (posterior shoulder and scapular muscles). Strength in these muscles will greatly aid your posture and assist you in preventing the rounded shoulders and tendency for "forward posturing". This also aids in maintaining the flexibility needed in your shoulders for activities of daily living, such as upper extremity dressing, bathing, and grooming.

Airplane

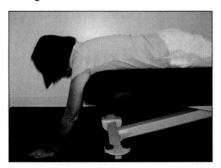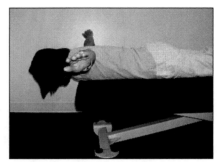

START POSITION: Lie flat on your stomach with your arms hanging down over the edge of your mat or bed.

ACTION/FINISH POSITION: Lift your arms out to the sides with your wrist, elbow and shoulders in the same plane as though you are flying like an airplane. Hold this position for 5 seconds and repeat to complete the desired amount of repetitions. Keep your head and neck neutral with your eyes gaze straight down. Do not gaze forward, because this will hyper-extend your neck.

PURPOSE: To stimulate the postural muscles in your upper back (posterior shoulder and scapular muscles). Strength in these muscles will greatly aid your posture and assist you in preventing the rounded shoulders and tendency for "forward posturing." This also aids in maintaining the flexibility needed in your shoulders for activities of daily living, such as upper extremity dressing, bathing, and grooming.

CHAPTER NINE

Level Three Exercises

LEVEL THREE: Mildly symptomatic (standing balance good, no assistive device)

This group will require the ability for good general balance without the need of upper extremity support. If you are able to walk without an assistive device, such as a cane, you should be able to perform the following exercises. If your balance is impaired to the level that does not allow you to safely perform the standing exercises, please proceed to level 2 exercise program. We recommend you start out with 1 set of 10 repetitions for each exercise and build up to performing 2-3 sets of 10 as you can tolerate it. We suggest that you also break up the exercises into different days so that you are not performing such a large volume of exercises at one time. You may want to perform the sitting exercise on opposite days of the mat exercises. A good schedule may involve performing the sitting group on Monday, Wednesday, Friday and the mat exercise group on Tuesday and Thursday. The following week you can then reverse the days. We also recommend that you limit your time to spending 20-30 minutes maximum per exercise session. It is much better to get into the habit of exercising daily for 15-20 minutes than to skip days then to do too much to make up for missing days.

SUGGESTED EXERCISE LIST:

Standing Exercise routine
1) Wall standing arm raise

2) Wall standing arm diagonals

3) Wall standing alternate arm/leg lift

4) Standing squats

5) Lunges

Mat exercise routine
1) Bridges with leg lifts

2) Lower Trunk Rotation

3) Supermans

4) Airplanes

5) Alternating Arm/Leg lifts on stomach

STANDING WALL EXERCISES

The standing exercises will require the ability for general balance without the need of upper extremity support. If you are able to walk without an assistive device, you should be able to perform the following exercises. If your balance is impaired to the level that does not allow you to safely perform the standing exercises, please proceed to the sitting and mat exercises.

Wall standing arm raise

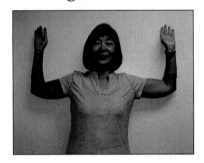 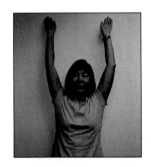

START POSITION: Stand with heels, buttocks, shoulders and head against a wall. Bring your arms up so that your elbows, bent at 90 degrees, are at the same level as your shoulders.. Maintain as much contact of your arms with the wall as possible.

ACTION/FINISH POSITION: Squeeze your shoulder blades together and maintain full contact with the wall as you slowly raise your arms overhead until they are completely straight. Hold this position for 10 seconds and slowly return back to the start position.

PURPOSE: To stimulate and work the postural muscles as you move your arms. This exercise also promotes stability of your scapular muscles which will assist in maintaining functional strength and range of motion in your arms for activities of daily living.

Wall Standing Diagonals

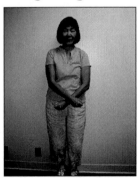 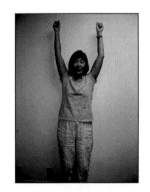

START POSITION: Stand with heels, buttocks, shoulders and head against wall with each hand over the opposite hip.

ACTION/FINISH POSITION: Maintain contact with the wall during the exercise. Squeeze your shoulder blades together while lifting your arms simultaneously in a diagonal position until your arms are extended and straightened overhead.

PURPOSE: To stimulate and work the postural muscles as you move your arms. This exercise also promotes stability of your scapular muscles which will assist in maintaining functional strength and range of motion in your arms for activities of daily living.

Wall Standing alternating arm-leg lift

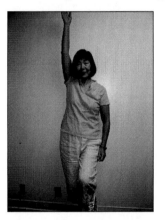 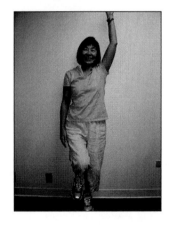

START POSITION: Stand with heels, buttocks, shoulders and head against a wall.

ACTION/FINISH POSITION: While maintaining contact with the wall, purposely shift your weight to the right leg and lift the left leg while you simultaneously raise your right arm. Return to the start position and repeat by alternating lifting your opposite arm/leg.

PURPOSE: To stimulate and work the postural muscles as you shift weight and move your legs. This exercise promotes good posture while you move dynamically and trains you in "anti-freezing techniques" by consciously, purposely engaging in controlled movement.

Standing squats

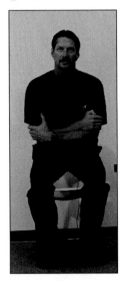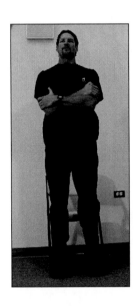

START POSITION: Sit with arms forward across chest.

ACTION/FINISH POSITION: Bend forward at your hips until your nose is past your toes. Push up with your legs while keeping your head and shoulders in front of your feet until you are standing tall/erect. If you cannot perform with arms folded, you can use your hands to assist in pushing up.

PURPOSE: To stimulate and work the postural muscles, in particular hip extensors (gluteals) and knee extensors (quadriceps).

Standing Lunges

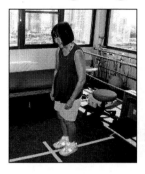 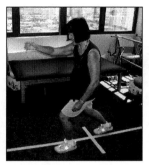 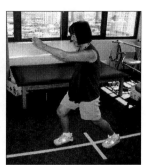

START POSITION: Stand with feet even.

ACTION/FINISH POSITION: Lunge forward with one leg while maintaining the position of the opposite leg back. Return to the start position and repeat with the other leg.

PURPOSE: To stimulate and work the postural muscles, in particular hip extensors (gluteals) and knee extensors (quadriceps), as well as challenging balance.

MAT EXERCISES

The mat exercises do not require very much balance and are appropriate for everyone as long as you can achieve the required positions. The positions that may be the most difficult to achieve are those requiring you to lie on your stomach. The focus of mat exercises is the same as the wall exercises, to encourage purposeful movement and to strengthen the postural muscles to better combat the forward posturing and other related PD symptoms.

Bridges alternate leg lift

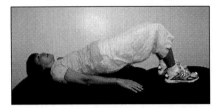 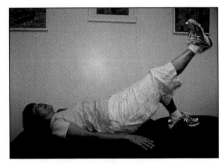

START POSITION: Lie down on your back with your arms extended at your sides. Bend both of your knees so that your feet are flat on the mat or bed.

ACTION/FINISH POSITION: Hold your stomach tight as you squeeze your buttocks muscles and lift your buttocks as high off the mat or bed as possible. Hold the bridge position while you extend your right leg and hold for 5 seconds. While still maintaining the bridge return the right leg to the mat and repeat on left side, all while still maintaining the bridge. Return to the start position and then repeat for the desired amount of repetitions.

PURPOSE: This exercise focuses on the postural muscles for hip and back extension as well as core strengthening. Your hip and back extensors will aid you in maintaining the strength and motion for a more upright posture.

Lower trunk rotation (wind shield washers)

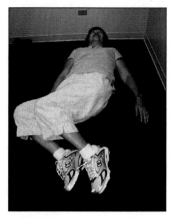 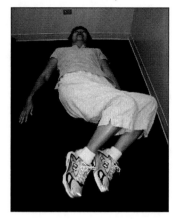

Beginning

START POSITION: Lie down on your back with your arms at your sides. Bend both of your knees so that your feet are flat on the mat or bed.

ACTION/FINISH POSITION: Maintain your shoulders in contact with the bed during the entire exercise. While keeping your knees and feet together, roll your knees as far to the right as possible (You will feel a stretch on the opposite side). Hold for 3 seconds and then roll your knees as far as possible to the left side. Return to the start position and then repeat for the desired amount of repetitions.

PURPOSE: This exercise focuses on trunk rotation. Flexibility in your trunk or pelvic rotation is essential for maintaining an efficient walking pattern as well as general mobility, such as getting in and out of a car or out of bed.

Superman

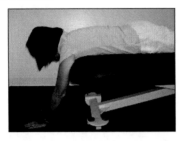 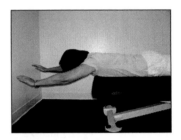

START POSITION: Lie flat on your stomach with your arms hanging down over the edge of your mat or bed.

ACTION/FINISH POSITION: Lift your arms straight up in front of you as high as you can, as if you are flying like superman. Hold this position for 5 seconds and repeat to complete the desired amount of repetitions. Keep your head and neck neutral with your gaze straight down. Do not look forward because this will hyper-extend your neck.

PURPOSE: To stimulate the postural muscles in your upper back (posterior shoulder and scapular muscles). Strength in these muscles will greatly aid your posture and assist you in preventing the rounded shoulders and tendency toward "forward posturing." This also aids in maintaining the flexibility needed in your shoulders for activities of daily living, such as upper extremity dressing, bathing, and grooming.

Airplane

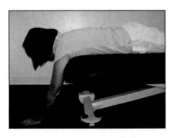 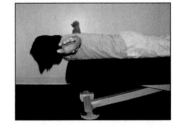

START POSITION: Lie flat on your stomach with your arms hanging down over the edge of your mat or bed.

ACTION/FINISH POSITION: Lift your arms out to the sides with your wrists, elbows, and shoulders in the same plane, as though you are flying like an airplane. Hold this position for 5 seconds and repeat to complete the desired amount of repetitions. Keep your head and neck neutral with your gaze straight down. Do not look forward because this will hyper-extend your neck.

PURPOSE: To stimulate the postural muscles in your upper back (posterior shoulder and scapular muscles. Strength in these muscles will greatly aid your posture and assist you in preventing the rounded shoulders and tendency toward "forward posturing". This also aids in maintaining the flexibility needed in your shoulders for activities of daily living, such as upper extremity dressing, bathing, and grooming.

Alternate leg/arm lifts on stomach

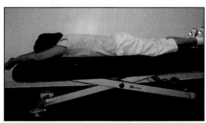 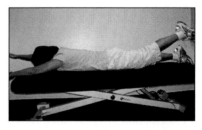

START POSITION: Lie flat on your stomach with your arms and legs fully extended.

ACTION/FINISH POSITION: Purposely shift your weight to the right side and lift the left leg, while you simultaneously raise your right arm. Return to the start position and repeat by alternately lifting your opposite arm/leg.

PURPOSE: To stimulate and work the postural muscles as you shift weight to off-load your opposite leg. This exercise promotes good posture as it stimulates nearly all of your extensor or "anti-gravity" postural muscles.

CHAPTER TEN

Community Gym

The type and models of exercise equipment in a community fitness setting will vary greatly. This list is far from being all inclusive. What we are presenting in this section are some common pieces of equipment that may be appropriate for combating your PD symptoms.

Row

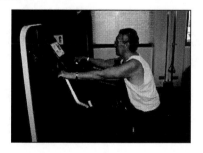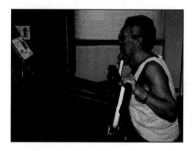

Beginning

START POSITION: Adjust the seat so your shoulders are level with the handles. Adjust the arm pad so your arms are fully extended when grasping the handles with your palms facing down.

ACTION/FINISH POSITION: Apply the appropriate weight. Without moving your torso, pull the handles backwards while leading with your elbows. Bring the elbows behind the shoulders, pause and slowly return to the start position.

PURPOSE: To stimulate the postural muscles in your upper back (posterior shoulder and scapular muscles). Strength in these muscles will greatly aid your posture and assist you in preventing the rounded shoulders and tendency toward "forward posturing". This also aids in maintaining the flexibility needed in your shoulders for activities of daily living, such as upper extremity dressing, bathing, and grooming.

Lat-Pulldown

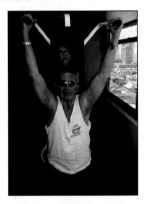 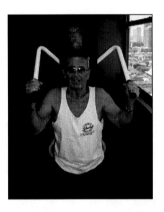

START POSITION: Adjust the seat so your feet are securely on the floor. Apply the appropriate weight. Stand and grasp in a palm down position. Sit down while maintaining your arms fully extended overhead.

ACTION/FINISH POSITION: Pull the handles downward leading with your elbows until your elbows are below your shoulders, pause and slowly return to the starting position.

PURPOSE: To stimulate the postural muscles in your upper back as well as strengthening the primary stabilizer of the upper spine (latisimus dorsi). This also aids in maintaining the flexibility needed in your shoulders for activities of daily living, such as upper extremity dressing, bathing, and grooming.

Torso-Rotary

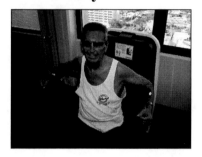 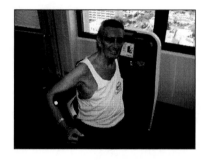

START POSITION: Adjust the seat so your feet are securely on the floor. Apply the appropriate weight. Set rotator stop to the appropriate angle.

ACTION/FINISH POSITION: Starting from the left, rotate the trunk as far as is possible and comfortable to the right. Slowly return to start position. Perform desired number of repetitions and repeat alternately rotating to the left.

PURPOSE: This particular exercise is excellent in general but especially for PD because it promotes trunk rotation, which can aid in combating trunk rigidity. Often the loss of arm swing on one side and loss of trunk rotation are the first gait (walking) symptoms or deviations that occur.

Shoulder Press

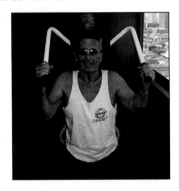 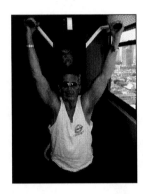

Beginning

START POSITION: Adjust the seat so the hand grips are parallel to your shoulders. Apply the appropriate weight. Sit with head, back, and buttocks against the back support.

ACTION/FINISH POSITION: Push the handles straight up and overhead. Once arms are fully extended, pause and lower weight. Slowly return to the start position. Perform desired number of repetitions and repeat to the opposite side.

PURPOSE: This particular exercise promotes shoulder strength and flexibility, which can aid in activities of daily living. It also promotes symmetry and a greater midline orientation of trunk.

Leg press

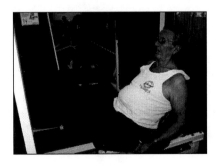

START POSITION: Apply the appropriate weight. Sit in the machine with your back flat against the support and your hips at a 90 degree angle to your trunk. Place your feet shoulder width apart on the foot plate.

ACTION/FINISH POSITION: Push the foot plate forward by extending your knees and hips. Slowly return to the start position. Make a conscious effort to push equally with both legs, especially if you feel that one leg has more PD symptoms; otherwise, you may end up working the lesser affected leg much more which could lead to muscle soreness.

PURPOSE: To stimulate and work the postural muscles, in particular the hip extensors (gluteals) and knee extensors (quadriceps).

Leg Extension

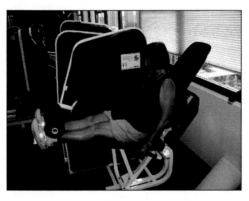

START POSITION: Adjust the seat or backrest so the front edge of the seat cushion is 1-2" behind your knee joint. Adjust the shin pad to be just above your ankle. Apply the appropriate weight. Sit with head, back, and buttocks against the back support.

ACTION/FINISH POSITION: Straighten your knees to full extension. Slowly return to start position. Perform desired number of repetitions and repeat to the opposite side.

PURPOSE: This particular exercise promotes full knee extension. It is common for persons with PD to walk with their hips and knees flexed. The quadriceps (knee extensors) are one of the muscle groups that are anti-gravity in nature and promote a more upright posture. Quadricep strength is also a key indicator of mobility and fall risk. Studies show that persons with normal quadricep strength are at lower risk for falls and have increased mobility over those who suffer weakness.

CHAPTER ELEVEN

Flexibility

As mentioned earlier, flexibility is important for maintaining good posture, safe walking, and the ability to perform your activities of daily living, such as dressing. These benefits illustrate the importance of including stretching for flexibility in an exercise routine. Optimizing your flexibility can allow you more efficient movement that will enhance mobility.

The areas that need the most attention are your hip flexors, knee flexors, as well as your anterior chest and shoulders. Maintaining the ability to stand up straight with full hip and knee extension can aid in reducing fatigue and decrease the tendency toward forward posturing and a leaning, festinating walking pattern. If your knees and hips are fully extended, your body is mechanically stacked requiring less effort. Once you stand and walk in a flexed posture, you are asking your muscles to work much harder, which leads to fatigue.

In addition to your legs and hips, maintaining good shoulder range of motion will not only aid in balance but also maintain the ability to perform activities of daily living. One of the first complaints I hear from my female patients is the loss of the ability to manage their bra. Many times this is due to loss of range of motion, not just decreasing hand dexterity.

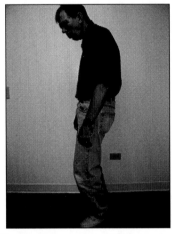

Illustrates a typical PD posture

When Should I Stretch?

You should not just jump in and start stretching your cold muscles. Like an old car in the winter, your muscles require some time to warm up. Elevated body temperatures tend to improve the ability to perform physical work. Gentle physical activity allows the blood to circulate to the muscles and tendons, which warms them up and makes them more pliable. This will reduce the potential risk of stretching-induced injuries.

Simple warm-up activities can include rolling your shoulders forward and backward and slow wheelchair propulsion. Arm circles, clockwise and counterclockwise, are also excellent general activities to warm up the whole arm. If you are going to perform leg exercises, walking may be useful to increase the circulation to the working muscles of your legs. Gentle riding on a stationary bicycle for 3 to 5 minutes is also a good activity. Once you have increased the circulation to your working muscles, you can perform gentle static stretching to prepare your muscles for your workout.

Principles of Stretching

Static Stretching

Static stretching is the preferred mode of stretching for most individuals because if done properly there is little risk of injury. Static means that the stretch is held constant for a certain range of motion around one or a sequence of joints.

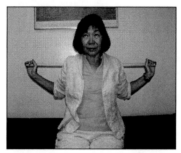

Example of a static stretch for the anterior shoulders and chest.

Frequency

Stretching exercises need to be performed daily to maintain flexibility. Whole-body stretching is necessary to maintain functional range of motion so you can perform the activities of daily living, even if you are non-ambulatory. For example, if you use a wheelchair for locomotion, stretching your legs may not relate to wheelchair propulsion but it can assist with proper positioning in your wheelchair and with the ability to get the lower half of your body dressed.

Intensity

In regard to stretching, intensity refers to how much tension is produced by the stretch. The degree of stretch can be increased or decreased by the amount of time the stretch is held and the amount of external force applied to produce the stretch. The tension produced should not cause pain—pain means you have pushed too far. There should be no pain when you stretch; you should feel slight tension that slowly diminishes with the stretch. Apply stretches gradually, building to a maximum as the tissues release, and then remove the stretch gradually to prevent rebound or tightening of the muscle.

Duration

How long you hold a stretch contributes to the intensity. Static stretches should be maintained for 30 to 60 seconds. Your goal is to change the resting length of a muscle tissue and tendon, so the bottom line is the longer you hold the stretch at your end range of motion, the better.

BASIC STRETCHING RULES

- No bouncing. Hold static stretching to build up soft tissue tension so change can occur in tissue length. Bouncing can tear tissues or cause injuries in other affected areas.

- No pain. Stretching should not cause a sensation of discomfort or tension; pain indicates that you have pushed too far.

- Do not hold your breath. Exhale with short-duration stretches and breathe slowly and rhythmically with longer duration stretches so you are relaxed and focused on the muscles you are stretching.

- Know what you are stretching and why. Each individual and sport has different flexibility requirements; individual assessments are required to recognize tight and unstable areas.
  Watch for muscle substitution and make sure the proper group is being stretched.

Precautions with Stretching

If you have any of the following conditions, check with a physician or physical therapist before implementing a flexibility routine. You need to be knowledgeable about the structural stability of your bones, joints, and muscles and understand restrictions or precautions that you may need to follow, with both stretching and exercise. For example, if you have a history of joint laxity at the knee, you may have to wear a knee brace to help control this laxity during stretching and exercise.

These conditions require professional clearance:

1. Severe spasticity with resultant joint contractures; the presence of a joint contracture or deformity

2. The diagnosis of osteoporosis or heterotopic ossification

3. A history of joint laxity (hypermobility), or joint subluxation (partial dislocation), or joint dislocation

4. A surgical history with resulting scar tissue, tissue adhesions, joint fusions, or placement of instrumentation to stabilize a fracture

5. Pain that limits movement or has yet to be evaluated by a physician or physical therapist

No Stretching: Contraindications for Stretching

The following existing conditions indicate that a stretching routine should not be performed at all or only by a medical professional. These conditions need to be evaluated and monitored by a medical professional to prevent injury:

1. An infection in an extremity or joint

2. Excessive swelling in a joint

3. Severe, painful joint crepitus

4. An open wound in the area you want to stretch

5. The onset of pain in an extremity

6. New joint instability or laxity that has yet to be evaluated by a physician or physical therapist

Flexibility Exercises
The Door Way Stretch

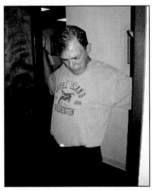

Hold on to both sides of a doorway with your hands behind you at ear level. Lean into the doorway to stretch the chest and anterior shoulder. Hold stretch for a minimum of 30 seconds and repeat as needed.

Behind the back pull

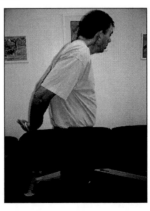

Clasp your hands behind your back, lift your arms up until you feel a stretch in the anterior shoulder and chest. Keep your chest out and chin tucked. Try not to bend forward at the hips during this exercise. Hold the stretch for a minimum of 30 seconds. Repeat as needed.

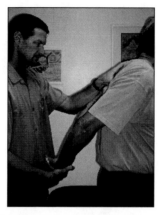

Illustrates the "Behind the Back Pull Stretch" with slight over pressure from a partner for a greater stretch.

Above the Head Reach Stretch

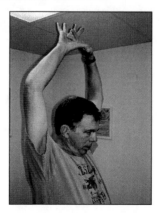

Grasp one hand over the other above your head with palms facing upward. Push your arms up to stretch the anterior and inner arm. Hold the stretch for a minimum of 30 seconds. Repeat as needed.

Behind the Head Cane Pull

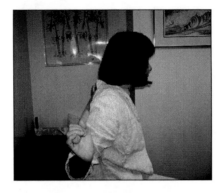

Lift a cane or broomstick horizontally with both hands in a wide grasp. Bring it over and behind your head and attempt to move it down as far as it will go without pushing your head forward. Hold the stretch for a minimum of 30 seconds and repeat as needed. This is a stretch for your chest and anterior shoulders.

Chicken Wing Stretch

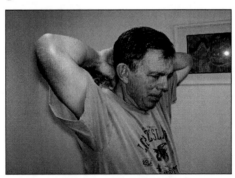

Place your hands behind your head with your fingers clasped. Try not to push your head forward. Squeeze your shoulder blades while pressing your elbows backwards. Hold the stretch for a minimum of 30 seconds and repeat as needed. This is a stretch for your chest and anterior shoulders.

Back and Hip Extension Stretch

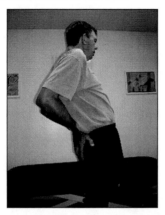

Place your hands on your hips and extend your upper trunk backwards while pushing your hips forward and keeping your knees straight. Hold the stretch for a minimum of 30 seconds and repeat as necessary. This is a stretch for your hip flexors.

Prone Lying on Elbows

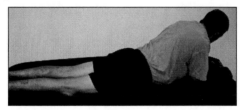

Lying on your stomach and keeping your hips on the supporting surface, place your hands just above the shoulder level and slowly push up to stretch the abdominals and hip flexors.

Supine Stretcher

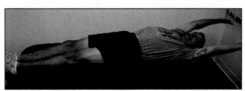

Lie flat on your back with your legs completely flat on the supporting surface. Reach your arms up and over your body as far as they will go. Hold this position for a minimum of 30 seconds and repeat as needed. This position stretches all of your anterior muscles which tend to get tight.

Lower Trunk Rotation Stretch

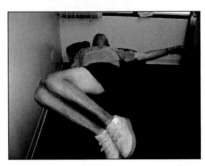

Lie on your back with your knees bent and feet flat on the mat or bed. Roll your knees off to the right while reaching with your left arm to the left. Hold this stretch for a minimum of 30 seconds and repeat in the opposite direction.

Seated Hamstring Stretch

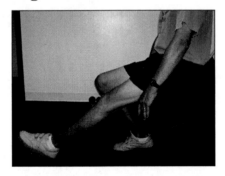

Sitting at the edge of a chair, place one leg straight out with the heel resting on the floor. Apply gentle pressure to the knee to keep it extended and lean the trunk forward, maintaining an erect back, to stretch hamstrings. You should feel a pulling sensation in the back of your knees and thigh. Hold the stretch for a minimum of 30 seconds. Repeat as needed.

Partner Hamstring Stretch

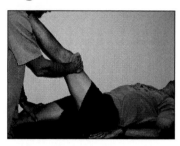

As you lie on your back, a helper will lift one leg without bending the knee while keeping the other leg flat on the mat. You should feel a pulling sensation in the back of your knees and thigh. Hold the stretch for a minimum of 30 seconds. Repeat as needed.

Gastroc & Soleus (Calf) Stretch

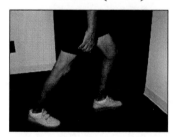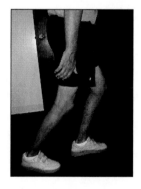

Stand in a stride position with one leg ahead of the other. Keep the heel of the back leg down as you lean forward towards the front leg, while your back leg is straight. This stretches the gastroc muscle. Hold for a minimum of 30 seconds. To stretch the soleus muscle, perform the same position as above but bend the knee of your back leg.

ABOUT THE AUTHOR

Kevin Lockette, PT

Kevin has been practicing as a physical therapist in the rehabilitation field since 1989. He is the primary author of a medical text on rehabilitation, ***Conditioning with Physical Disabilities, Human Kinetic Publishers 1994*** and has written numerous articles and lectured extensively in the areas of exercise with emphasis on physical disabilities.

Kevin has extensive experience in acute rehabilitation and is the founder of what is now one of the nation's largest wellness programs for individuals with physical disabilities at the renown Rehabilitation Institute of Chicago. Kevin is a past head coach for the United States Disable Sports Team (A member of the U.S. Olympic Committee) and coached in International games including the World Championships and the Paralympics in Barcelona, Spain in 1992. Kevin is presently on the Clinical Advisory Council for the Multiple Sclerosis Society-Hawaii as well as a founding member of Hawaii's Parkinson Disease Center of Excellence.

Kevin enjoys canoe paddling and weight lifting. He is also an avid college basketball fan and attends UH sports whenever he can. Kevin is not only a physical therapist, but also the father of two, an athlete, and a nonfiction history buff. He is musically inclined in the harmonica and ukelele with a love for the blues.

APPENDIX

Home assessment checklist

PROBLEM	ENTRY SOLUTION	NOTES
☐ unable to safely negotiate stairs ☐ risers too high ☐ nosings catching foot ☐ open riser catching foot ☐ slipping on stairs ☐ need balance support ☐ difficulty distinguishing edges or thresholds	☐ ramp ☐ add rails ☐ bevel nosing ☐ close risers ☐ non-slip treads: stairs/ramp ☐ chair lift ☐ mark edge of each tread with distinguishing strip ☐ change ramp slope ☐ increase lighting	

PROBLEM	DOORS SOLUTION	NOTES

☐ Too narrow for passage
☐ Landing too small to manage door w/wheelchair or assistive device
☐ Thresholds – tripping hazard or a barrier
☐ Door mats – tripping hazard
☐ Marking/wear on door
☐ Difficulty managing door handle
☐ Difficulty managing lock
☐ Door swing hazard (interior door)
	☐ Swing clear hinges (adds 1 ½ to 1 ¾ in. on the thickness of the door)
	☐ Remove door stops (adds ¾ in.)
	☐ Remove door
	☐ Automatic door opener
	☐ Enlarge landing
	☐ Replace door
	  ☐ sliding
	  ☐ folding
	  ☐ pocket
	  ☐ swing (widen)
	☐ Remove threshold
	☐ Change threshold to lower profile
	☐ Beveled ramp for threshold
	☐ Secure door mat
	☐ Recess to be flush (new construction)
	☐ Add kick-plates
	☐ Lever adapter for cylinder knob
	☐ Lever hardware (door knob)
	☐ Loop hardware (door knob)
	☐ Slide bolts
	☐ Relocate lock
	☐ Vision panels	

PROBLEM	BATHROOM SOLUTION	NOTES
☐ Sink ☐ no clearance under sink for wheelchair ☐ too low – bending difficulty ☐ limited hand dexterity	☐ Remove sink cabinet doors ☐ cover pipes (insulation) ☐ add decorative curtains ☐ Remove cabinet wall mounts ☐ cover pipes (insulation) ☐ add decorative curtains ☐ Raise sink/vanity ☐ Lower sink/vanity ☐ Replace knobs with single lever faucet ☐ Replace knobs with double levers or cross knobs	

☐ Toilets
  ☐ seat too high
  ☐ seat too low
  ☐ difficulty with toilet
    transfer
☐ Shower/Tub
  ☐ transfer to tub
    unsafe
  ☐ inability to stand or
    decreased balance
    in tub
	☐ Raised toilet seat
	☐ Footstool
	☐ Grab bars
	  ☐ wall mount
	  ☐ sheltering arms
	  ☐ pivoting
	☐ Tub seat
	☐ Tub transfer bench
	☐ Tub chair
	☐ Hand held shower
	☐ Tub lifts
	☐ Add non-skid
	  surface
	☐ Add wall-mount
	  grab bars
	☐ Add removable tub
	  grab bars
	☐ Roll in shower
	☐ Transfer shower
	☐ Shower chair
	☐ Anti-scald
	  temperature controls	

Appendix

	☐ Install emergency call button or telephone, or make sure the nearest existing telephone can be safely brought into bathroom ☐ Make sure mirror and medicine cabinet are easy to use, bottom edge of mirror should be no higher than 42 in. from floor; install tilting mirror ☐ Install heat lamp ☐ Install ceiling vent fan	

107

PROBLEM	KITCHEN SOLUTION	NOTES
☐ Difficulty accessing freezer	☐ Side by side refrigerator/freezer	

☐ Counter/Work surface
  ☐ too high
  ☐ too low
  ☐ no wheelchair clearance underneath
  ☐ impaired hand dexterity
	☐ Stand alone table
	☐ Wheelchair lap board
	☐ Folding/pullout shelves
	☐ Wood boards across drawers
	☐ Remove base cabinets
	☐ Remove cabinet drawers
	☐ Spiked cutting boards
	☐ Replace/add counters, locate according to specific needs
	  ☐ adjustable
	  ☐ manual
	  ☐ electric
	☐ Add "hot item" shelf to or adjacent to the oven	

☐ Sink
  ☐ too deep
  ☐ no clearance under sink for wheelchair
	☐ Install rack
	☐ Remove cabinet doors
	☐ Remove cabinet/wall mount sink
	☐ Hand held hose/ sprayer	

☐ Cook top
   ☐ wheelchair user cannot reach back burners
   ☐ difficult visibility for cooking
   ☐ difficulty moving pots and pans full of water or food
☐ Wheelchair access limited with standard [over below?] stove
	☐ Staggered burners
	☐ Add mirror above stove
	☐ Flush ceramic cook tops
	☐ Add wall mount over microwave	

☐ Storage/cabinets	☐ Replace storage drawer hardware with easy gliding hardware or simplify current operations, include "C" or "D" shaped handles ☐ Install "lazy susan" in corner cabinetry ☐ Consider open or pull-out shelves (open shelves above counter provide better storage for older consumers, especially if kept as low as possible); if not open shelves, consider transparent front for easy visibility to the inside ☐ Add towel rack, low shelves to cabinet doors ☐ Electric can opener, jar cover opener, grip enhancer, timer w/ large number, long-handle "reacher"	

PROBLEM	FLOORS SOLUTION	NOTES
	☐ Secure rug corners and edges, area rugs can help define areas ☐ Cover potentially slippery floors with textured runners, carpet ☐ Use vinyl, rubber, cork floor tile ☐ Use non-glare material ☐ Use heavyweight, high-density, short pile, level carpet	

PROBLEM	LIGHTING SOLUTION	NOTES

	☐ Install fixtures at locations that resident uses most often, or place lamps adjacent to most used locations
	☐ Use light fixtures with more than one bulb/increase light bulb wattage
	☐ Light switches at door to each room
	☐ Larger rocker switches
	☐ Locate switches and thermostats no higher than 48 inches above floor (specific location depending on specific needs)
	☐ Pain switches a contrasting color to wall
	☐ Put locator lights on switches
	☐ Add a *strobe* light on door bell
	☐ Use light dimmer switches
	☐ Install stair light
	☐ Use blinds or shades to control glare from outdoor light
	☐ Light colored walls tend to give more light
	☐ If glare is a problem, use textured wall paper or matte paint finishes on walls
	    ☐ Use color to define an area or to heighten contrast between objects or areas including where the wall meets the floor
	    ☐ Locate electric outlets higher than standard height, ideally at least 27 inches from the floor	

PROBLEM	STORAGE SOLUTION	NOTES
	☐ Use track sliding doors (possibly tracks on top and bottom); bi-fold doors are also easy to use ☐ Use roll-out drawers or other drawers with easy to use hardware ☐ Use dual-height clothes rails or adjustable rods (possibly a rotating carousel) ☐ Rearrange storage for maximum usefulness given potential reaching, stretching, and bending limitations	

ORGANIZATION LINKS

National Parkinson Foundation, Inc.: www.parkinson.org

The American Parkinson Disease Association, Inc.: www. apdaparkinson.com/

Parkinson's Action Network :http://www.parkinsonsaction.org

Colorado Neurological Institute http://www.thecni.org/ movementdisorders

Michael J. Fox Foundation for Parkinson's Research - http://www. michaeljfox.org

Movers & Shakers Inc.: http://www.pdadvocates.org

Northwest Parkinson's Foundation: http://www.nwpf.org

Parkinson Association of the Carolinas: http://www. parkinsonassociation.org

Parkinson Society Canada : http://www.parkinson.ca

Parkinson's Disease Foundation: http://www.pdf.org

Parkinson's Foundation of Out Reach Care & Encouragement: http://www.pforce.org

PLWP, Inc - People Living With Parkinson's: http://www.plwp.org

Re-Wired For Life : http://www.rewiredforlife.org

Awakenings: http://www.parkinsonsdisease.com

Ability: Parkinson's Disease: http://www.ability.org.uk/parkinso. html

Meditopia: http://meditopia.com/dis/park/otpark.html

Parkinson's Disease Interest Group: http://www.santel.lu/santel/ diseases/parkins.html

BIBLIOGRAPHY

Palmer SS, Mortimer JA, Webster DD, Bistevins R, Dickinson GL.
Exercise therapy for Parkinson's disease.
Arch Phys Med Rehabil. 1986 Oct;67(10):741-5.

Scandalis TA, Bosak A, Berliner JC, Helman LL, Wells MR.
Resistance training and gait function in patients with Parkinson's disease.
Am J Phys Med Rehabil. 2001 Jan;80(1):38-43; quiz 44-6.

Cakit BD, Saracoglu M, Genc H, Erdem HR, Inan L.
The effects of incremental speed-dependent treadmill training on postural instability and fear of falling in Parkinson's disease.
Clin Rehabil. 2007 Aug;21(8):698-705.

Reuter I, Engelhardt M, Stecker K, Baas H.
Therapeutic value of exercise training in Parkinson's disease.
Med Sci Sports Exerc. 1999 Nov;31(11):1544-9.

Nelson AJ, Zwick D, Brody S, Doran C, Pulver L, Rooz G, Sadownick M, Nelson R, Rothman J.
The validity of the GaitRite and the Functional Ambulation Performance scoring system in the analysis of Parkinson gait.
NeuroRehabilitation. 2002;17(3):255-62.

Herman T, Giladi N, Gruendlinger L, Hausdorff JM.
Six weeks of intensive treadmill training improves gait and quality of life in patients with Parkinson's disease: a pilot study.
Arch Phys Med Rehabil. 2007 Sep;88(9):1154-8.

Crizzle AM, Newhouse IJ.
Is physical exercise beneficial for persons with Parkinson's disease?
Clin J Sport Med. 2006 Sep;16(5):422-5. Review.

Miyai I, Fujimoto Y, Ueda Y, Yamamoto H, Nozaki S, Saito T, Kang J.
Abstract
Treadmill training with body weight support: its effect on Parkinson's disease.
Arch Phys Med Rehabil. 2000 Jul;81(7):849-52.

Viliani T, Pasquetti P, Magnolfi S, Lunardelli ML, Giorgi C, Serra P, Taiti PG.
Abstract
Effects of physical training on straightening-up processes in patients with Parkinson's disease.
Disabil Rehabil. 1999 Feb;21(2):68-73.

Hackney ME,Kantorovich S, Levin R, Earhart GM. Effects of *Tango on Mobility in Parkinson's Disease: Preliminary Study. J* Neurol. Physical therapy 2007 Dec; 31 (4) 173-9.